NCLEX-RN®
DRUG GUIDE

Seventh Edition

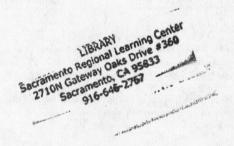
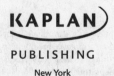

KAPLAN

PUBLISHING

New York

© 2017 by Kaplan, Inc.

Published by Kaplan Medical, a division of Kaplan, Inc.
750 Third Avenue
New York, NY 10017

10 9 8 7 6 5 4 3 2 1

ISBN: 978-1-5062-2347-6

Kaplan Publishing print books are available at special quantity discounts to use for sales promotions, employee premiums, or educational purposes. For more information or to purchase books, please call the Simon & Schuster special sales department at 866-506-1949.

TABLE OF CONTENTS

Additional resources available at

www.kaptest.com/nclexrnbookresources

TEN STEPS FOR MASTERING THE DRUGS ON THE NCLEX-RN EXAM

The best way to use this book to study for your nursing boards is to have a specific plan of attack! Then you can approach the sizeable task of learning about medications with confidence.

1. Get your mind set for future success.

Focus on the fact that, after you pass the NCLEX and become a licensed registered nurse (*not* "if you pass"), you will be using the information you learned in this book in your daily life, both personal and work.

You will be using drug information every day. Likewise, you need to study these go-to meds every day, even if it's only in short bursts. Don't rely on your previous experience of passing exams by pulling exhausting all-nighters. Do picture your study as gaining a solid understanding of concepts useful for your entire career.

2. Understand the book's flashcard format.

Think of the arrangement of information in this book as your two-sided master slide templates.

Medication category

Medication subcategory

GENERIC NAME

(phonetic pronunciation guide)

(Brand/Trade Name)

Purpose: why the drug is given for a specifc set of diseases or clinical conditions

---

Front flashcard information

On the right-hand page, medications are arranged alphabetically under 22 drug categories. Each category tells which body system or medical condition the drug targets. Subcategories group drugs with similar desired action within that body system or for that medical condition.

For example, the first drug category, "Allergy and Asthma Medications," divides 11 medications under the following headings:

- Antihistamines (5 meds listed alphabetically by generic name)
- Corticosteroids (6 meds listed alphabetically by generic name)

To build a firm mental connection between medication facts, talk to yourself! First, pronounce the generic name while looking at the phonetic pronunciation guide. Then, say the generic name again, while looking at the medication category and subcategory. Engaging 3 learning channels at once (looking, talking, and listening) promotes active learning and enhances your recall.

SIDE EFFECTS

First side effect

Second side effect, etc.

NURSING CONSIDERATIONS

- Information about drug pharmacodynamics (how the human body responds to a drug) and pharmacokinetics (how a drug behaves in the human body)
- Other nursing considerations
- Key patient education highlights
- Rx or OTC (or both); controlled substance schedule (if applicable)

Back flashcard information

The nursing profession is about action. Therefore, the most critical nursing implications for you to learn can be summarized as "go" or "no go" decisions for 2 situations:

- A vital sign such as pulse or respirations directs the nurse to withhold a medication (such as: no digoxin if the patient's pulse is under 60 beats per minute).
- A specific side effect signals a medical condition that is severe enough to warrant calling the health care provider immediately.

3. Keep your focus on the medication triangle.

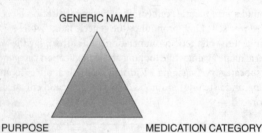

GENERIC NAME

PURPOSE   MEDICATION CATEGORY

Knowing the *purpose* for which the medication is designed allows you to accurately match patient and drug. It firmly links the drug to the mental connections you established connecting the *generic name* with the *medication category*.

4. Calendar in chunks of time for formal study.

Plan on spending time with this book—but it doesn't have to happen all at once! This book is designed to be studied piecemeal. For example, if you want to review the whole book over 3 weeks, plan on a chapter a day. That lets you read the 22 chapters one drug category at a time.

5. Consider both paper and people companionship.

This small book has purposely been sized to fit into a purse or pocket. Take it with you everywhere you go—think of it as your new, rectangular BFF.

Waiting in line can become an opportunity to review one drug category. Counting down the minutes until the microwave rings is enough time to look at another drug category.

If you know a fellow student who is as motivated as you are, talk to them about setting up a "buddy system" where you can review your latest learning for each other. Make it a game: Quiz each other, *Jeopardy!* style, with one person giving the generic name and the other person guessing the purpose of that medication. You may be surprised by how these games energize you to prepare and remember.

6. Record your progress and thoughts.

By keeping track of your steps forward, you will enjoy 2 benefits: remembering where you left off, and marking the milestones of your journey. When you feel confident that you can recall the information up to a certain point in the book, mark it in some way that signals to you, "Done."

Make your messages to yourself obvious. What will communicate "Read here" or "Completed!" to you—a handwritten note? Folding over the corner of each completed page? Check marks in the margins? Remember: This is your book. Personalize it to work best for *you*.

Other additions that may help you focus on the material: circling or underlining key words, using a highlighter to enliven the facts you need with bright color, or mapping out similarities and differences of comparable medications in hand-drawn diagrams or tables. The more you interact with the material, the better you will be able to apply it.

7. Be alert for drug groupings.

The same suffix used in 2 or more medications hints at similarities in drug category and subcategory. Take the hint! As you go through the book, be alert for these "family" groupings, and chart them in your active study. Here is an example you can follow:

Suffix	Drug Category	Drug Subcategory	Generic Names
–afil	Genitourinary	Erectile dysfunction	Sildenafil Tadalafil Vardenafil
–asone	Allergy and asthma	Corticosteroids	Beclomethasone Fluticasone Mometasone
–azosin	Cardiovascular	Alpha blockers	Doxazosin Prazosin Terazosin
–cillin	Anti-infectives	Penicillins	Amoxicillin Ampicillin Penicillin
–dipine	Cardiovascular	Calcium channel blockers	Amlodipine Felodipine Nifedipine
–olol	Cardiovascular	Beta blockers	Atenolol Metoprolol Propranolol
–pam	Mental health	Antianxiety	Diazepam Lorazepam Citalopram

Suffix	Drug Category	Drug Subcategory	Generic Names
–pril	Cardiovascular	ACE inhibitors	Benaze**pril** Capto**pril** Enala**pril** Lisino**pril** Rami**pril**
–romycin	Anti-infectives	Macrolides	Azith**romycin** Clarith**romycin** Eryth**romycin**
–statin	Cardiovascular	Antilipemic	Atorva**statin** Fluva**statin** Lova**statin** Prava**statin** Rosuva**statin** Simva**statin**
–tidine	Gastrointestinal	Antiulcer	Cime**tidine** Famo**tidine** Rani**tidine**
–vir	Anti-infectives	Antiviral	Acyclo**vir** Oseltami**vir** Valacyclo**vir**

8. Don't worry about brand names.

You are unlikely to see any trade/brand names on your NCLEX. The National Council of State Boards of Nursing, Inc., which develops the exam, strives for consistency over time—a stance that favors either the generic name or the drug category/subcategory. Trade and brand names are at the discretion of the many pharmaceutical manufacturing companies that produce them. *Trade and brand names can change.* Generic names are more stable, and thus are favored by the National Council.

9. Take a quick final review.

Shortly before Test Day, pick up this book once again. Even if you only have the opportunity to look at the table of contents, doing so will refresh your memory before you take the NCLEX.

10. Get ready to celebrate!

Once you've passed the exam, keep this book as a souvenir of that fact that you earned your place in the ranks of registered nurses!

CETIRIZINE HCL
(se-<u>teer</u>-a-zeen)

(Zyrtec)

Purpose: relief of seasonal allergic rhinitis symptoms

• •

DIPHENHYDRAMINE
(dye-fen-<u>hye</u>-dra-meen)

(Benadryl)

Purpose: relief of allergy symptoms, rhinitis, and motion sickness; nighttime sedation

SIDE EFFECTS

Drowsiness   Headache
Dry mouth   Constipation

NURSING CONSIDERATIONS

- Relief of perennial allergic rhinitis caused by molds, animal dander, and other allergens
- Avoid alcohol during cetirizine therapy
- Call provider immediately for difficulty breathing or swallowing
- Notify provider for hydroxyzine (Vistaril) allergy
- Rx

• •

SIDE EFFECTS

Dizziness, drowsiness   Nausea, diarrhea   Photosensitivity
Palpitations,   Dysuria   Chest tightness,
  hypotension   Urinary retention   wheezing
Blurred vision   Thrombocytopenia

NURSING CONSIDERATIONS

- Take with meals for GI symptoms; absorption rate may slightly decrease
- Take at bedtime only if using as sleep aid
- PO: peak 2–4 hours
- IM: onset 30 minutes, peak 2–4 hours
- Should be discontinued 4 days before skin allergy tests
- Avoid driving and other hazardous activities if drowsiness occurs
- Avoid use of alcohol, CNS depressants
- Rx

FEXOFENADINE
(fex-oh-<u>fen</u>-a-deen)

(Allegra)

Purpose: management of rhinitis and allergy symptoms

• •

HYDROXYZINE
(hye-<u>drox</u>-i-zeen)

(Atarax, Vistaril)

Purpose: treatment of pruritus, pre-op anxiety, and post-op nausea/ vomiting; potentiation of opioid analgesics and sedation

SIDE EFFECTS

Drowsiness	Diarrhea	Itching
Headache	Vomiting	Hoarseness
Dizziness	Rash	Urinary retention

NURSING CONSIDERATIONS

- Avoid alcohol, CNS depressants
- Notify provider if taking erythromycin or ketoconazole (Nizoral)
- If taking aluminum magnesium antacid, take antacid a few hours before or after fexofenadine
- Rx

· ·

SIDE EFFECTS

Drowsiness	Headache
Dry mouth, nose, and throat	Chest congestion
Dizziness	

NURSING CONSIDERATIONS

- PO: onset 15–30 minutes, duration 4–6 hours
- Avoid use with alcohol, CNS depressants
- Treatment of symptoms of alcohol withdrawal
- Notify provider of diagnosis of glaucoma, ulcers, enlarged prostate gland, liver disease, hypertension, seizures, or hyperthyroidism
- Rx

Allergy and Asthma Medications
Antihistamines

LORATADINE
(lor-<u>a</u>-ti-deen)

(Alavert, Claritin)

Purpose: management of seasonal rhinitis

· ·

Allergy and Asthma Medications
Corticosteroids

BECLOMETHASONE
(be-kloe-<u>meth</u>-a-sone)

(Beclovent, Beconase)

Purpose: treatment of chronic asthma and of seasonal and perennial rhinitis

SIDE EFFECTS

Headache	Rash
Dry mouth	Stomach pain
Diarrhea	Tachycardia

NURSING CONSIDERATIONS

- Avoid alcohol, CNS depressants
- Take on empty stomach 1 hour before or 2 hours after meals
- Onset 1–3 hours, peak 8–12 hours, duration ≥ 24 hours
- OTC, Rx

• •

SIDE EFFECTS

Hoarseness	Headache	Rhinitis
Oropharyngeal fungal infections	Sore throat	Cough
	Dyspepsia	Angioedema

NURSING CONSIDERATIONS

- Prevention of recurrence of nasal polyps after surgical removal
- Nasal spray: onset 5–7 days (up to 3 weeks in some patients), peak up to 3 weeks
- Inhaler: onset 10 minutes
- Use regular peak flow monitoring to determine respiratory status
- Rinse mouth after each use to prevent oral fungal infections
- Rx

FLUNISOLIDE
(floo-<u>niss</u>-oh-lide)

(Aerobid, Nasalide)

Purpose: treatment of chronic asthma and of seasonal and perennial rhinitis

• •

FLUTICASONE
(floo-<u>tik</u>-a-sone)

(Flonase)

Purpose: treatment of chronic asthma and of seasonal and perennial rhinitis

SIDE EFFECTS

Dysphonia

Hoarseness

Oropharyngeal
  fungal infections

Headache

Sore throat

Nasal congestion,
  cold symptoms

Nausea, vomiting,
  diarrhea

Epistaxis
  (nosebleed)

NURSING CONSIDERATIONS

- Onset: few days
- Use regular peak flow monitoring to determine respiratory status
- Rx

• •

SIDE EFFECTS

Hoarseness

Oropharyngeal
  fungal infections

Headache

Nasal congestion,
  cold symptoms

Nausea, vomiting,
  diarrhea

Epistaxis
  (nosebleed), nasal
  irritation

Dyspnea

NURSING CONSIDERATIONS

- Nasal spray: onset within 2 days, peak 1–2 weeks
- Use regular peak flow monitoring to determine respiratory status
- Rx

FLUTICASONE PROPIONATE SALMETEROL

(floo-<u>tik</u>-a-sone <u>proe</u>-pee-oh-nate sal-<u>meh</u>-te-role)

(Advair Diskus)

Purpose: treatment of asthma that is not well controlled with long-term corticosteroids; treatment of COPD

• •

MOMETASONE

(moe-<u>met</u>-a-sone)

(Nasonex Spray)

Purpose: treatment of chronic asthma and of seasonal or perennial rhinitis

SIDE EFFECTS

Nausea, vomiting, diarrhea

Headache

Hoarseness

Oropharyngeal fungal infections

Muscle and bone pain

Viral respiratory infections, bronchitis

NURSING CONSIDERATIONS

- Oral inhalation; rinse mouth with water after inhalation
- Twice-daily dosage, 12 hours apart; used long term
- Use regular peak flow monitoring to determine respiratory status
- Monitor growth of pediatric patient
- May decrease bone mineral density
- Monitor for eosinophilic conditions, hypokalemia, and hyperglycemia
- Rx

• •

SIDE EFFECTS

Hoarseness

Oropharyngeal fungal infections

Headache

Sore throat

Nasal congestion, cold symptoms

Nausea, vomiting, diarrhea

Muscle or joint pain

NURSING CONSIDERATIONS

- Nasal spray: onset few days, peak up to 3 weeks
- Use regular peak flow monitoring to determine respiratory status
- Rx

TRIAMCINOLONE
(try-am-<u>sin</u>-oh-lone)

(Nasacort AQ Spray)

Purpose: treatment of chronic asthma and of seasonal or perennial rhinitis

• •

Analgesics
Nonopioid Analgesics

ACETAMINOPHEN
(a-seet-a-<u>min</u>-a-fen)

(Tylenol)

Purpose: treatment of mild pain or fever

SIDE EFFECTS

Agitation

Oropharyngeal fungal infections

Headache

Blurred vision

Nausea, vomiting, diarrhea

Increased cough

Bronchitis

NURSING CONSIDERATIONS

- Nasal spray: onset few days, peak 3–4 days
- PO/IM: peak 1–2 hours
- Use regular peak flow monitoring to determine respiratory status
- Rx

• •

SIDE EFFECTS

Anemia (long-term use)

Liver and kidney failure

Dyspnea (prolonged high
  doses)

Angioedema

Hives, itching

NURSING CONSIDERATIONS

- PO: onset less than 1 hour, peak 30 minutes to 2 hours, duration 4–6 hours
- Rectal: onset slow, peak 1–2 hours, duration 3–4 hours
- Take crushed or whole with full glass of water
- Can give with food or milk to decrease GI upset
- Signs of chronic poisoning: rapid, weak pulse; dyspnea; cold, clammy extremities
- Signs of chronic overdose: bleeding, bruising, malaise, fever, sore throat, anorexia, jaundice
- OTC

ACETAMINOPHEN/ASPIRIN/CAFFEINE
(a-seet-a-<u>min</u>-a-fen/<u>as</u>-pir-in/kaf-<u>een</u>)

(Excedrin)

Purpose: treatment of mild to moderate pain or fever

· ·

ASPIRIN
(<u>as</u>-pir-in)

Purpose: management of mild to moderate pain or fever and TIA; prophylaxis of MI, ischemic stroke, and angina

SIDE EFFECTS

Upset stomach, heartburn
Depressed mood, anxious or restless feelings
Insomnia

NURSING CONSIDERATIONS

- Do not give to children or teenagers with fever, flu symptoms, or chickenpox; Reye syndrome may develop
- Watch out for symptoms of stomach bleeding or liver problems

· ,

SIDE EFFECTS

Nausea, vomiting	Tinnitus
Rash	GI bleeding
Dyspnea	

NURSING CONSIDERATIONS

- PO: onset 15–30 minutes, peak 1–2 hours, duration 4–6 hours
- Rectal: onset slow, 20%–60% absorbed if retained 2–4 hours
- With long-term use, check for liver damage: dark urine, clay-colored stools, yellowing of skin and sclera, itching, abdominal pain, fever, diarrhea
- For arthritis, give 30 minutes before exercise; may take 2 weeks before full effect is felt
- Discard tablets if vinegar-like smell
- Do not give to children or teens with flulike symptoms or chickenpox; Reye syndrome may develop
- OTC

CELECOXIB
(sel-eh-<u>cox</u>-ib)

(Celebrex)

Purpose: management of acute chronic arthritis pain, relief of primary dysmenorrheal pain within 60 minutes

• •

IBUPROFEN
(eye-byoo-<u>proe</u>-fen)

(Advil, Motrin IB)

Purpose: treatment of mild to moderate pain, reduction of inflammation

SIDE EFFECTS

Fatigue

Anxiety, depression, nervousness

Nausea, vomiting, anorexia, dry mouth, constipation

Dyspnea

Back pain

Tachycardia

Dysuria

Palpitations

NURSING CONSIDERATIONS

- Onset: 24–48 hours, duration 12–24 hours
- Can take without regard to meals
- Do not take if allergic to sulfonamides, aspirin, or NSAIDs
- Rx

. . . .

SIDE EFFECTS

Headache

Tinnitus

Nausea, anorexia

Dizziness

Blood dyscrasias

Constipation

GI bleeding

NURSING CONSIDERATIONS

- Treatment of rheumatoid arthritis, osteoarthritis, primary dysmenorrhea, gout, dental pain, musculoskeletal disorders, fever
- Onset: 30 minutes, peak 1–2 hours
- Take with food or milk to decrease GI symptoms
- Contact provider if ringing or roaring in ears, which may indicate toxicity
- Contact provider if changes in urinary pattern, increased weight, edema, increased pain in joints, fever, or blood in urine, which may indicate kidney damage
- Use sunscreen to prevent photosensitivity
- Avoid use with ASA, NSAIDs, and alcohol, which may precipitate GI bleeding
- Avoid use with anticoagulants
- OTC, Rx

NAPROXEN
(na-<u>prox</u>-en)

(Aleve [OTC], Naprosyn)

*Purpose: treatment of mild to moderate pain, reduction of
inflammation*

• •

TRAMADOL
(<u>tram</u>-a-dole)

(Ultram, Ultram ER)

Purpose: management of moderate to severe pain and chronic pain

SIDE EFFECTS

GI bleeding
Blood dyscrasias
Tinnitus
Insomnia

Vision changes
Rash
Angioedema
Jaundice

Tachycardia
Nausea, vomiting, diarrhea

NURSING CONSIDERATIONS

- Treatment of rheumatoid, juvenile, and gouty arthritis; osteoarthritis; primary dysmenorrhea
- Patients with asthma, ASA hypersensitivity, or nasal polyps have increased risk of hypersensitivity
- Contact provider if blurred vision or ringing or roaring in ears, which may indicate toxicity
- Contact provider if black stools, flulike symptoms
- Contact provider if changes in urinary pattern, increased weight, edema, increased pain in joints, fever, or blood in urine, which may indicate kidney damage
- Avoid use with ASA, steroids, and alcohol
- May increase risk of MI or stroke
- OTC, Rx

• •

SIDE EFFECTS

Dizziness, confusion
Headache
Orthostatic hypotension
Abnormal ECG

Visual disturbances
Nausea, vomiting
GI bleeding
Urinary retention/ frequency

Rash
Respiratory depression

NURSING CONSIDERATIONS

- Give with antiemetic for nausea, vomiting
- Take without or without food
- May cause serotonin or neuroleptic malignant syndrome–like reactions
- Avoid OTC medications unless approved by provider
- Rx

BUPRENORPHINE/NALOXONE
(byoo-pra-<u>nor</u>-feen / na-<u>lox</u>-own)

(Suboxone)

*Purpose: management of severe pain, treatment of opioid
  dependence*

• •

CODEINE
(<u>koe</u>-deen)

*Purpose: treatment of moderate to severe pain and of nonproductive
  cough*

SIDE EFFECTS

Drowsiness
Sleepiness
Itching, rash
Blurred vision

Palpitations,
   tachycardia
Headache
Mental changes

Hepatotoxicity
Respiratory
   depression

NURSING CONSIDERATIONS

- Avoid hazardous activities until reaction known
- Avoid alcohol and CNS depressants
- IM: onset 15 minutes, peak 1 hour
- IV: onset 1 minute, peak 5 minutes
- SL: onset and peak unknown
- Rx C-V (parenteral), C-III (tablet)

• •

SIDE EFFECTS

Drowsiness, sedation
Nausea, vomiting, anorexia
Respiratory depression
Constipation
Orthostatic hypotension

Dysuria
Dyspnea
Seizures
Bradycardia

NURSING CONSIDERATIONS

- PO: onset 30–45 minutes, peak 60–120 minutes, duration 4–6 hours
- IM/subQ: onset 10–30 minutes, peak 30–60 minutes, duration 4–6 hours
- Do not give if respirations are less than 12 per minute
- Avoid use with alcohol, CNS depressants
- Withdrawal symptoms may occur: nausea, vomiting, cramps, fever, faintness, anorexia
- Physical dependency may result from long-term use
- Rx C-II, III, IV, V (depends on route)

HYDROCODONE/ACETAMINOPHEN

(hye-droe-<u>koe</u>-doan/a-seet-a-<u>min</u>-a-fen)

(Lortab, Vicodin)

Purpose: treatment of moderate to severe pain

• •

HYDROMORPHONE

(hye-droe-<u>mor</u>-fone)

(Dilaudid)

Purpose: treatment of moderate to severe pain and of nonproductive cough

SIDE EFFECTS

Dizziness
Drowsiness
Constipation
Nausea
Vomiting
Respiratory depression

Sedation
Impairment of mental and
   physical performance
Rash
Pruritus
Palpitations

NURSING CONSIDERATIONS

- Use with CNS depressants and/or alcohol may result in addictive CNS depression
- May be habit-forming
- Avoid alcohol during treatment
- Use with caution in patients with pulmonary considerations
- Rx C-III

• •

SIDE EFFECTS

Drowsiness, sedation
Nausea, vomiting, anorexia
Respiratory depression
Constipation, cramps

Orthostatic hypotension
Confusion, headache
Rash

NURSING CONSIDERATIONS

- PO: onset 15–30 minutes, peak 30–60 minutes, duration 4–6 hours
- IM: onset 15 minutes, peak 30–60 minutes, duration 4–5 hours
- IV: onset 10–15 minutes, peak 15–30 minutes, duration 2–3 hours
- subQ: onset 15 minutes, peak 30–90 minutes, duration 4 hours
- Rectal: duration 6–8 hours
- Do not give if respirations are less than 12 per minute
- Avoid use with alcohol, CNS depressants
- Withdrawal symptoms may occur: nausea, vomiting, cramps, fever, faintness, anorexia
- Physical dependency may result from long-term use
- Elderly patients may require lower doses
- Rx C-II

MEPERIDINE
(me-<u>pair</u>-i-deen)

(Demerol)

Purpose: treatment of moderate to severe pain

• •

METHADONE
(<u>meth</u>-a-doan)

(Dolophine, Methadose)

Purpose: treatment of severe pain, detoxification/management of narcotic addiction

SIDE EFFECTS

Drowsiness, sedation
Respiratory depression
Orthostatic hypotension
Confusion, headache

Euphoria
Bradycardia
Diaphoresis
Urticaria

NURSING CONSIDERATIONS

- PO: onset 10–15 minutes, peak 30–60 minutes, duration 2–4 hours (usually 3)
- IM: onset 10–15 minutes, peak 30–50 minutes, duration 2–4 hours (usually 3)
- IV: onset less than 5 minutes, peak 5–7 minutes, duration 2–4 hours (usually 3)
- subQ: onset 10–15 minutes, peak 30–50 minutes, duration 2–4 hours (usually 3)
- Do not give if respirations are less than 12 per minute
- Avoid use with alcohol, CNS depressants
- Withdrawal symptoms may occur: nausea, vomiting, cramps, fever, faintness, anorexia
- Physical dependency may result from long-term use
- Do not co-infuse with barbiturates, aminophylline, heparin, morphine, methicillin, phenytoin, sodium bicarbonate, sulfadiazine, or sulfisoxazole
- Rx C-II

• •

SIDE EFFECTS

Drowsiness, sedation
Nausea, vomiting, anorexia

Respiratory depression
Constipation, cramps
Orthostatic hypotension

Confusion, headache
Rash
Arrhythmias
Agitation

NURSING CONSIDERATIONS

- PO: onset 30–60 minutes, peak 30–60 minutes, duration 4–6 hours (with continuous dosing, duration of action may increase to 22–48 hours)
- Do not give if respirations are less than 12 per minute
- Avoid use with alcohol, CNS depressants
- Withdrawal symptoms may occur: nausea, vomiting, cramps, fever, faintness, anorexia
- Physical dependency may result from long-term use
- Rx C-II

MORPHINE
(<u>mor</u>-feen)

(MS Contin)

Purpose: treatment of severe pain

• •

OXYCODONE
(ox-i-<u>koe</u>-doan)

(OxyContin; with aspirin Percodan, with acetaminophen Percocet)

Purpose: treatment of moderate to severe pain

SIDE EFFECTS

Respiratory depression
Sedation

Euphoria
Orthostatic hypotension

Bradycardia
Diaphoresis
Urticaria

NURSING CONSIDERATIONS

- Continuous dosing is more effective than prn; may be given by patient-controlled analgesia (PCA)
- PO: onset 15–60 minutes, peak 30–60 minutes, duration 3–6 hours
- IM: onset 10–15 minutes, peak 30–50 minutes, duration 2–4 hours (usually 3)
- IV: onset less than 5 minutes, peak 18 minutes, duration 3–6 hours
- subQ: onset 10–15 minutes, peak 30–50 minutes, duration 2–4 hours (usually 3)
- Withdrawal symptoms may occur: nausea, vomiting, cramps, fever, faintness, anorexia
- Physical dependency may result from long-term use
- Monitor for increased respiratory and CNS depression when given with cimetidine, clomipramine, nortriptyline, or amitriptyline
- Rx C-II

• •

SIDE EFFECTS

Drowsiness, sedation
Nausea, vomiting, anorexia
Respiratory depression

Constipation
Confusion, headache
Rash
Euphoria

Urinary retention
Orthostatic hypotension
Palpitations

NURSING CONSIDERATIONS

- PO: peak 30–60 minutes, duration 4–6 hours
- Controlled-release: peak 3–4 minutes, duration 12 hours
- Do not give if respirations are less than 12 per minute
- Avoid use with alcohol, CNS depressants
- Withdrawal symptoms may occur: nausea, vomiting, cramps, fever, faintness, anorexia
- Physical dependency may result from long-term use
- Rx C-II (controlled-release) (Percocet)

DABIGATRAN ETEXILATE
(da-bi-<u>ga</u>-tran e-<u>tex</u>-i-late)

(Pradaxa)

Purpose: prevention of stroke in patients with nonvalvular atrial fibrillation

• •

ENOXAPARIN
(ee-noks-a-<u>par</u>-in)

(Lovenox)

Purpose: prevention and treatment of deep vein thrombosis

SIDE EFFECTS

Dyspepsia

Abdominal discomfort

Epigastric pain

GI hemorrhage

Bleeding

NURSING CONSIDERATIONS

- PO: may take without regard to meals
- Do not crush or chew capsules
- Closely monitor for signs of bleeding
- Increased risk of bleeding when combined with aspirin, other antiplatelets, or anticoagulants
- Stop med 24 hours before surgery
- Rx

• •

SIDE EFFECTS

Bleeding

Bruising

Injection site hematoma

Injection site ecchymosis

Increase in AST/ALT

NURSING CONSIDERATIONS

- Injection: subQ; can be given IV during cardiac procedures
- Do not use in patients with a history of heparin-induced thrombocytopenia
- Use with caution in patients with impaired renal function or morbid obesity
- Monitor closely for signs of bleeding or excessive bruising
- Stop med 12–24 hours before surgery
- Rx

HEPARIN
(<u>hep</u>-a-rin)

Purpose: prevention and treatment of deep vein thrombosis and pulmonary embolism

• •

Anticoagulants
Anticoagulants

RIVAROXABAN
(riv-a-<u>rox</u>-a-ban)

(Xarelto)

Purpose: treatment and prevention of deep vein thrombosis and pulmonary embolism, prevention of stroke in patients with nonvalvular atrial fibrillation

SIDE EFFECTS

Spontaneous bleeding	Anemia
Tissue irritation/pain at injection site	Thrombocytopenia
	Fever
Increased AST/ALT	Rash

NURSING CONSIDERATIONS

- Therapeutic PTT @ 1.5–2.5 times the control without signs of hemorrhage
- IV: peak 5 minutes, duration 2–6 hours (give over 1 minute)
- Injection: give deep subQ; never IM (danger of hematoma), onset 20–60 minutes, duration 8–12 hours
- Antidote: protamine sulfate within 30 minutes
- Assess for signs of hemorrhage
- Avoid ASA-containing products and NSAIDs
- Wear medical information tag
- Abrupt withdrawal may precipitate increased coagulability
- Rx

• •

SIDE EFFECTS

Bleeding	Syncope	Elevated bilirubin
Bruising	Nausea	Elevated ALT/AST
Pruritus	Hematoma	

NURSING CONSIDERATIONS

- Dose reduction required in renal impairment
- PO: give doses greater than 15 mg with food; lower doses may be given without regard to food
- Stop med 24 hours before surgery
- Monitor closely for signs of bleeding or excessive bruising
- Rx

WARFARIN
(<u>war</u>-far-in)

(Coumadin)

Purpose: prevention and treatment of deep vein thrombosis and pulmonary embolism, treatment of atrial fibrillation

• •

CARBAMAZEPINE
(kar-ba-<u>maz</u>-e-peen)

(Carbatrol, Tegretol)

Purpose: management of seizures, trigeminal neuralgia, and neuropathic pain

SIDE EFFECTS

Hemorrhage	Angina syndrome	Elevated liver enzymes
Diarrhea	Anemia	
Rash	Dermatitis	Anaphylactic reactions
Fever	Jaundice	

NURSING CONSIDERATIONS

- Therapeutic PT @ 1.5–2.5 times the control, INR @ 2.0–3.0
- Onset: 12–24 hours, peak 1.5–3 days; duration 3–5 days
- Avoid foods high in vitamin K: many green leafy vegetables
- Do not interchange brands; potencies may not be equivalent
- Do not take any drug or herb without provider approval—may change effect
- Avoid ASA-containing products and NSAIDs
- Oral anticoagulants may cause red-orange discoloration of alkaline urine, interfering with some lab tests
- Wear medical information tag
- Antidote: vitamin K
- Rx

• •

SIDE EFFECTS

Myelosuppression	Photosensitivity	Aplastic anemia
Dizziness, drowsiness	Depression	Stevens-Johnson syndrome
Ataxia	Nausea	Suicidal thoughts
Diplopia, rash	Vomiting	
	Dyspepsia	

NURSING CONSIDERATIONS

- Avoid driving and other activities requiring alertness the first 3 days
- Monitor blood levels, CBC regularly, esp. during first 2 months; periodic eye exams
- Take with food or milk to decrease GI upset
- Do not mix with grapefruit juice
- Urine may turn pink to brown
- Avoid abrupt withdrawal; discontinue gradually
- Avoid use with alcohol, CNS depressants
- Inform provider before taking any new medication or herbal medication
- Rx

CLONAZEPAM
(kloe-<u>naz</u>-uh-pam)

(Klonopin)

Purpose: management of seizures and panic disorder

• •

DIVALPROEX SODIUM
(dye-<u>val</u>-proe-ex)

(Depakote, Depakote ER)

Purpose: management of seizures, prophylaxis of migraine headache

SIDE EFFECTS

Drowsiness, dizziness

Behavioral changes

Poor coordination

Palpitations, tachycardia

Blurred vision

Increased salivation

Nausea, constipation

Dysuria

Libido changes

Thrombocytopenia

Respiratory depression

Rash

Muscle weakness

NURSING CONSIDERATIONS

- Do not discontinue abruptly, seizures may increase
- Avoid alcohol, CNS depressants
- May take with food or milk to decrease GI symptoms
- Report signs of toxicity: bone marrow suppression, nausea, vomiting, ataxia, diplopia, cardiovascular collapse
- May increase risk of suicidal thoughts
- Wear medication identification tag
- Rx C-IV

● ●

SIDE EFFECTS

Sedation, drowsiness, dizziness

Mental status and behavioral changes

Prolonged bleeding time

Nausea, vomiting, constipation, diarrhea

Hepatotoxicity

Teratogenicity

Pancreatitis

Thrombocytopenia

Headache

Diplopia

Alopecia

Multiorgan hypersensitivity

Rash

NURSING CONSIDERATIONS

- Take with or immediately after meals to lessen GI upset; swallow whole
- Avoid abrupt withdrawal after long-term use; discontinue gradually to prevent convulsions
- Monitor blood levels, platelets, bleeding time, and liver function tests
- Delayed-release products: peak blood level 3–5 hours, duration 12–24 hours
- Extended-release products: onset 2–4 days, peak blood level 7–14 hours, duration 24 hours
- Wear medical information tag
- Rx

GABAPENTIN
(<u>ga</u>-ba-pen-tin)

(Gabarone, Neurontin)

Purpose: management of seizures, postherpetic neuralgia, and primary restless leg syndrome

• •

LAMOTRIGINE
(la-<u>moe</u>-tri-jeen)

(Lamictal)

Purpose: management of seizures and bipolar disorder

SIDE EFFECTS

Drowsiness

Ataxia

Diplopia

Rhinitis

Constipation

Memory problems

Back or joint pain

Edema

Diarrhea

NURSING CONSIDERATIONS

- Do not take within 2 hours of antacid use
- Avoid abrupt withdrawal after long-term use; discontinue gradually over a week to prevent convulsions
- Give without regard to meals; can open capsules and put in juice or applesauce
- Do not crush or chew capsules
- Use caution with hazardous activities
- Wear medical information tag
- Rx

• •

SIDE EFFECTS

Ataxia, dizziness

Headache

Nausea, vomiting, anorexia

Rhinitis

Diplopia, blurred vision

Abdominal pain, dysmenorrhea

Loss of coordination

Mood changes

Irritability

Insomnia

Depression

NURSING CONSIDERATIONS

- In pediatric patients, stop at first sign of rash; all patients should notify provider of rashes
- Take divided doses with meals or just after to decrease adverse effects
- Use caution with hazardous activities until stabilized
- Avoid abrupt withdrawal; stop gradually to prevent increase in frequency of seizures
- Wear medical information tag
- Rx

MAGNESIUM SULFATE
(mag-<u>nee</u>-zee-um <u>sull</u>-fate)

*Purpose: prophylaxis of seizures that occur with preeclampsia;
treatment of eclampsia, acute nephritis in children, and
hypomagnesemia*

• •

PHENOBARBITAL
(fee-noe-<u>bar</u>-bi-tal)
(Luminal)

*Purpose: long-term management of seizures, management of febrile
seizures, therapeutic sedation*

SIDE EFFECTS

Muscle weakness
Flushing
Confusion, dizziness
Hypotension

Oliguria
Bradycardia
Decreased reflexes
Bradypnea

Hypophosphatemia
Hyperkalemia
Hypocalcemia

NURSING CONSIDERATIONS

- Given IM or IV
- Antidote: calcium gluconate
- Rx

• •

SIDE EFFECTS

Drowsiness,
  lethargy, rash
GI upset
Initially constricts
  pupils

Respiratory
  depression
Ataxia
Nightmares

Excitement in
  children
Dizziness
Hypotension
Thrombocytopenia

NURSING CONSIDERATIONS

- IV: slow rate—resuscitation equipment should be available
- IM: inject deep into large muscle mass to prevent tissue sloughing, can give subQ, onset 10–30 minutes
- PO: onset 20–60 minutes, peak 8–12 hours, duration 6–10 hours
- Use caution with hazardous activities until stabilized; drowsiness usually diminishes after initial weeks of therapy
- Long-term use withdrawal symptoms: vomiting, sweating, abdomen/muscle cramps, tremors, and possibly convulsions
- Vitamin D supplements are indicated for long-term use
- Rx C-IV

PHENYTOIN
(<u>fen</u>-i-toyn)
(Dilantin)

Purpose: management of seizures

● ●

PREGABALIN
(pre-<u>gab</u>-a-lin)
(Lyrica)

Purpose: treatment of neuropathic pain, postherpetic neuralgia, and fibromyalgia

SIDE EFFECTS

Drowsiness, ataxia
Nystagmus
Blurred vision
Rash
Hypotension

Lethargy
GI upset
Gingival
  hypertrophy
Depression

Urine discoloration
Thrombocytopenia
Hyperglycemia

NURSING CONSIDERATIONS

- PO: take divided doses, with or immediately after meals, to decrease adverse effects
- IV administration may lead to cardiac arrest—have resuscitation equipment available; never mix in IV with any other drug or dextrose
- Avoid abrupt withdrawal to prevent convulsions
- Do not use antacids or antidiarrheals within 2 hours of med
- Use caution with hazardous activities until stabilized
- Wear medical information tag
- Rx

• •

SIDE EFFECTS

Dizziness, tiredness,
  weakness
Headache
Nausea, vomiting,
  constipation
Flatulence, bloating

Mental status and
  behavioral changes
Lack of coordination
Increased appetite,
  weight gain
Back pain

Angioedema
Blurred vision
Tremor, twitching
Hypoglycemia

NURSING CONSIDERATIONS

- Take around the same time every day, 2–3 times daily; full therapeutic effects may require 4 weeks
- Do not crush or chew
- Avoid abrupt withdrawal after long-term use; discontinue gradually
- Avoid use with alcohol
- Use caution in potentially hazardous activities
- May increase the risk of suicidal thoughts or behavior
- Rx

TOPIRAMATE
(toh-<u>pie</u>-ruh-mate)

(Topamax, Topiragen)

Purpose: management of seizures, prophylaxis and treatment of migraines

● ●

VALPROATE, VALPROIC ACID
(val-<u>proe</u>-ate, val-<u>proe</u>-ic)

(Depacon, Depakene, Stavzor)

Purpose: management of seizures, prophylaxis of bipolar disorder and migraine

SIDE EFFECTS

Dizziness, drowsiness, fatigue

Impaired concentration/memory

Nervousness, speech problems

Nausea, weight loss

Vision problems

Ataxia

Photosensitivity

Behavior problems, mood problems

Anorexia

NURSING CONSIDERATIONS

- Give without regard to meals
- Avoid abrupt withdrawal after long-term use; discontinue gradually to prevent seizures and status epilepticus
- Do not crush or chew
- Use caution with hazardous activities until stabilized
- Increase fluid intake to prevent formation of kidney stones
- Notify provider immediately if experiencing periorbital pain or blurred vision
- Wear medical information tag
- Rx

. . . .

SIDE EFFECTS

Sedation, drowsiness, dizziness

Mental status and behavioral changes

Nausea, vomiting, constipation, diarrhea, heartburn

Prolonged bleeding time

Hepatotoxicity

Pancreatitis

Rash

Hypo/hypertension

Visual disturbances

SIADH

Dyspnea

NURSING CONSIDERATIONS

- Avoid abrupt withdrawal after long-term use; discontinue gradually to prevent convulsions
- May be given with food to decrease GI irritation
- Monitor for suicidal thoughts or behavior
- Rx

SUMATRIPTAN
(soo-ma-<u>trip</u>-tan)

(Imitrex)

Purpose: acute treatment of migraines

· ·

AMIKACIN, GENTAMICIN, TOBRAMYCIN
(am-i-<u>kay</u>-sin, jen-ta-<u>mye</u>-sin, toe-bra-<u>mye</u>-sin)

(Amikin, Garamycin, Tobrex)

Purpose: treatment of severe systemic infections of CNS, respiratory system, GI tract, urinary tract, bone, skin, and soft tissues

SIDE EFFECTS

Burning, tingling
Dizziness, numbness
Flushing
MI
Hypo/hypertension
Throat and nasal discomfort

Vision changes
Abdominal discomfort
Weakness, myalgia
Chest tightness, pressure

NURSING CONSIDERATIONS

- PO: swallow tablets whole, take as soon as symptoms appear
- Transdermal: apply to dry intact skin, discard after folding in half
- Onset 10 minutes to 2 hours, peak 10–20 minutes
- Ingestion of tyramine-containing foods (pickled products, beer, preservatives, chocolate) and caffeine may precipitate headaches
- Not to be used for more than 3–4 migraines per month
- Rx

• •

SIDE EFFECTS

Use during pregnancy can
    result in bilateral congenital
    deafness
Ototoxicity
Nephrotoxicity

Neurotoxicity
Allergic reaction: fever,
    difficulty breathing, rash
Vertigo, tinnitus

NURSING CONSIDERATIONS

- IV over 30 minutes to 1 hour; IM by deep, slow injection, never subQ
- Careful monitoring of blood levels
- Check peak—2 hours after med given
- Check trough—at time of dose/prior to med
- Monitor for signs of superinfection (diarrhea, URI, coated tongue)
- Immediately report hearing or balance problems
- Encourage fluids to 8–10 glasses/day
- Rx

AMOXICILLIN/CLAVULANATE
(a-mox-i-<u>sill</u>-in/<u>klav</u>-yoo-la-nate)
(Augmentin)

Purpose: treatment of lower respiratory infections, sinus and skin infections, otitis media, pneumonia, and impetigo

• •

Anti-Infectives
Antifungals

AMPHOTERICIN B
(am-fuh-<u>tair</u>-i-sin)
(Abelcet, Amphotec, Fungizone)

Purpose: treatment of invasive fungal infections

SIDE EFFECTS

Headache, agitation
Insomnia
Nausea, diarrhea, vomiting
Increased liver enzymes
Oliguria

Vaginitis
Bone marrow suppression
Hypo/hyperkalemia
Hypernatremia
Respiratory distress

NURSING CONSIDERATIONS

- Shake suspension before administering each dose
- Can be mixed with drinks
- Give with meal to increase absorption and reduce GI effects
- Give at equal intervals around to the clock to maintain blood levels
- Discard unused suspension after 14 days
- Nephrotoxic with high doses
- Rx

• •

SIDE EFFECTS

Blood, kidney, heart, liver
  abnormalities
GI upset
Hypokalemia
Skin irritation and thrombosis
  if IV infiltrates
Rash

Fever, chills
Malaise
Hypotension
Headache
Nephrotoxicity
Ototoxicity

NURSING CONSIDERATIONS

- Do not mix with other drugs
- Monitor vital signs; report fever or change in function, especially nervous system
- Meticulous care and observation of injection site
- Potential benefits must be balanced against serious side effects
- Rx

FLUCONAZOLE
(floo-<u>kon</u>-uh-zol)

(Diflucan)

Purpose: treatment of vaginal, esophageal, and systemic candidiasis and of cryptococcal meningitis

• •

HYDROXYCHLOROQUINE
(hye-<u>drox</u>-ee-<u>klor</u>-uh-kween)

(Plaquenil)

Purpose: management of lupus erythematosus, rheumatoid arthritis, and malaria

SIDE EFFECTS

Nausea

Diarrhea

Headache

Hepatotoxicity

Abdominal pain

NURSING CONSIDERATIONS

- Prothrombin time is increased after warfarin usage
- Take missed dose as soon as noticed, but do not double dose
- Monitor glucose levels, especially in diabetics
- Rx

- -

SIDE EFFECTS

Eye disturbances

Photosensitivity

Hypotension

Nausea, vomiting

Dizziness

Skin changes

Anorexia

Headache

Ototoxicity

NURSING CONSIDERATIONS

- Peak 1–2 hours
- Take at the same time each day to maintain blood level
- Give with meats to decrease GI distress
- For malaria, prophylaxis should be started 2 weeks before
  exposure and continue for 4–6 weeks after leaving exposure area
- Rx

QUININE SULFATE

(<u>kwye</u>-nine)

(Qualaquin)

Purpose: treatment of malaria

. . . .

Anti-Infectives
Antiprotozoals

METRONIDAZOLE

(meh-troe-<u>nye</u>-da-zole)

(Flagyl, Flagyl ER)

Purpose: treatment of a wide variety of infections including trichomoniasis, giardiasis, and bacterial vaginosis

SIDE EFFECTS

Eye disturbances

Nausea, vomiting

Anorexia

Tachycardia

Hypotension

Thrombocytopenia

Tinnitus

NURSING CONSIDERATIONS

- Peak 1–3 hours
- Take at the same time each day to maintain blood level
- May increase digoxin levels
- Do not crush
- OTC, Rx

• •

SIDE EFFECTS

Headache

Dizziness

Nausea, vomiting,
   diarrhea

Abdominal cramps

Metallic taste

Darkened urine

Depression

Blurred vision

Neurotoxicity

NURSING CONSIDERATIONS

- IV: immediate onset, PO: peak 1–2 hours
- Treatment of both partners is necessary in trichomoniasis
- Do not drink alcohol or preparations containing alcohol during and 48 hours after use; disulfiram-like reaction can occur
- Rx

ISONIAZID
(eye-soe-<u>nye</u>-a-zid)

(INH)

Purpose: treatment and prevention of tuberculosis

• •

ACYCLOVIR
(ay-<u>sye</u>-kloe-veer)

(Zovirax)

Purpose: treatment of herpes and varicella

SIDE EFFECTS

Peripheral
  neuropathy
Liver damage
Nausea, vomiting

NURSING CONSIDERATIONS

- PO/IM: onset rapid, peak 1–2 hours, duration up to 24 hours
- Contact provider if signs of hepatitis: yellow eyes and skin, nausea, vomiting, anorexia, dark urine, unusual tiredness, or weakness
- Contact provider if signs of peripheral neuropathy: numbness, tingling, or weakness
- Monitor liver tests
- Do not skip or double doses
- Rx

• •

SIDE EFFECTS

Headache	Nephrotoxicity
Blood dyscrasias	Tremors
Nausea, vomiting, diarrhea	Lethargy
Thrombocytopenia purpura	

NURSING CONSIDERATIONS

- IV: onset immediate, peak immediate
- PO: absorbed minimally, onset unknown, peak 90 minutes
- Do not break, crush, or chew capsules
- PO: take without regard to meals with a full glass of water
- If dose is missed, take as soon as remembered, up to 1 hour before next dose
- Contact provider if sore throat, fever, and fatigue; could be signs of superinfection
- Rx

OSELTAMIVIR PHOSPHATE
(oss-el-<u>tam</u>-i-veer)

(Tamiflu)

Purpose: prevention and treatment of influenza

• •

VALACYCLOVIR HCL
(val-a-<u>sye</u>-kloe-veer)

(Valtrex)

Purpose: treatment of herpes zoster (shingles), genital herpes, herpes labialis (cold sores), and varicella

SIDE EFFECTS

Nausea	Headache
Vomiting	Fatigue
Dizziness	Cough

NURSING CONSIDERATIONS

- Used to treat uncomplicated acute flu symptoms in patients that are symptomatic for 2 days or less
- Should not be used as a substitute for influenza vaccinations
- May be taken without regard to meals
- Rx

• •

SIDE EFFECTS

Nausea, vomiting, diarrhea	Dizziness
Abdominal cramps	Dysmenorrhea
Headache	Thrombocytopenic purpura
Rash	Increased AST

NURSING CONSIDERATIONS

- Patients should drink plenty of fluids during treatment
- Avoid sexual contact when lesions are visible
- Rx

ZIDOVUDINE

(zye-<u>doe</u>-vyoo-deen)

(AZT, Retrovir)

Purpose: management of HIV infection, postexposure prophylaxis of HIV following needlestick

• •

CEPHALEXIN

(sef-a-<u>lex</u>-in)

(Keflex)

Purpose: treatment of upper and lower respiratory tract, urinary tract, skin, bone, and otitis media infections

SIDE EFFECTS

Fever, headache, malaise   Dyspepsia
Nausea, vomiting, diarrhea   Rash
Dizziness   Hepatomegaly
Insomnia

NURSING CONSIDERATIONS

- GI upset and insomnia resolve after 3–4 weeks
- PO: peak 30–90 minutes
- Check with provider before taking aspirin, acetaminophen, or indomethacin
- Rx

• •

SIDE EFFECTS

Diarrhea   Nephrotoxicity
Anaphylaxis   Dyspnea
Nausea   Thrombocytopenia
Rash   Elevated liver function tests
Headache

NURSING CONSIDERATIONS

- Peak 1 hour, duration usually 6 hours, but may be up to 12 hours with decreased renal function
- Take for 10–14 days to prevent superinfection
- Possible cross allergy to penicillin
- May cause false positive of urine glucose
- Rx

CEFUROXIME
(sef-yoor-<u>ox</u>-eem)

(Ceftin, Zinacef)

Purpose: treatment of lower respiratory tract, urinary tract, skin, bone, joint, and gonococcal infections and of septicemia and meningitis

• •

CEFDINIR
(<u>sef</u>-di-neer)

(Omnicef)

Purpose: treatment of acute exacerbations of chronic bronchitis, sinusitis, pharyngitis, otitis media, tonsillitis, and skin infections

SIDE EFFECTS

Nausea, vomiting, diarrhea

Headache

Rash

Elevated liver function tests

Nephrotoxicity

Thrombocytopenia

NURSING CONSIDERATIONS

- Take for 10–14 days to prevent superinfection
- May cause increased BUN and serum creatine
- May cause false positive urine glucose
- Possible cross allergy to penicillin
- Rx

• •

SIDE EFFECTS

Nausea, vomiting, diarrhea

Anorexia

Rash

Elevated liver function tests

Headache

Oral and vaginal candidiasis

Dizziness

Neurotoxicity

Thrombocytopenia

NURSING CONSIDERATIONS

- Take for 10–14 days to prevent superinfection
- Do not give antacids or iron supplements within 2 hours
- May cause false positive for urine glucose
- Possible cross allergy to penicillin
- Rx

CEFEPIME
(<u>sef</u>-e-peem)

(Maxipime)

Purpose: treatment of respiratory tract, urinary tract, skin, and bone infections

• •

Anti-Infectives
Fluoroquinolones

CIPROFLOXACIN
(sip-roe-<u>flocks</u>-a-sin)

(Cipro)

Purpose: treatment of infections caused by E. coli and other bacteria and of chronic bacterial prostatitis, acute sinusitis, and postexposure inhalation anthrax

SIDE EFFECTS

Nausea, vomiting, diarrhea
Anorexia
Elevated liver function tests
Rash

Headache
Dyspnea
Nephrotoxicity

NURSING CONSIDERATIONS

- IV: peak 30 minutes
- IM: peak 2 hours
- May cause false positive for urine glucose
- Possible cross allergy to penicillin
- Rx

• •

SIDE EFFECTS

Seizures
Headache, restlessness
Nausea, vomiting, diarrhea,
    abd. distress, flatulence

Rash
Photosensitivity
Tendon rupture, muscle tear
Increased liver function test

NURSING CONSIDERATIONS

- Contraindicated in children less than 18 years of age
- Take 2 hours before or 6 hours after antacid or iron preparation
- Avoid caffeine
- Encourage fluids to 2–3 L/day
- May cause false positive in opiate screening tests
- Do not infuse with other medications
- Rx

LEVOFLOXACIN
(lee-va-<u>flocks</u>-a-sin)

(Levaquin)

Purpose: treatment of infections such as acute sinusitis, acute chronic bronchitis, pneumonia, and anthrax and of infections of the urinary tract, kidney, prostate, and skin

• •

Anti-Infectives
Glycopeptides

VANCOMYCIN
(van-ka-<u>my</u>-sin)

(Vancocin)

Purpose: treatment of C. difficile, resistant staph infections, colitis, and staph enterocolitis; prophylaxis for endocarditis and dental procedures

SIDE EFFECTS

Headache, nausea, vomiting, diarrhea

Stomach pain

Dizziness

Vaginal itching and/or discharge

Tendon rupture or tendinitis

Insomnia

Photosensitivity, rash

Hallucination, paranoia

Hepatotoxicity

Suicidal thoughts

Encephalopathy

Chest pain, palpitations

NURSING CONSIDERATIONS

- Infused injection over 60–90 minutes, once every 24 hours
- Monitor blood sugar; may cause hypoglycemia or hyperglycemia
- Rx

• •

SIDE EFFECTS

Nephrotoxicity

Headache

Ototoxicity

Dyspnea

NURSING CONSIDERATIONS

- PO: poor absorption
- IV: peak 5 minutes, duration 12–24 hours
- Give at least 60 minutes (IV); do not infuse with other drugs
- Give antihistamine if "red man syndrome": decreased blood pressure, flushing of face and neck
- Contact provider if signs of superinfection (sore throat, fever, fatigue)
- Check peak: 1 hour after infusion
- Check trough before next dose
- Encourage fluids to 2 L/day
- Rx

CLINDAMYCIN HCL PHOSPHATE
(<u>klin</u>-da-my-sin)

(Cleocin HCL, Cleocin Phosphate for IM)

Purpose: treatment of infections caused by Staphylococcus, Streptococcus, *and other bacteria*

· ·

AZITHROMYCIN
(a-zi-thro-<u>my</u>-sin)

(Zithromax)

Purpose: treatment of mild to moderate infections of the respiratory tract and skin and of nongonococcal urethritis, cervicitis, acute pharyngitis/tonsillitis, and community-acquired pneumonia

SIDE EFFECTS

Nausea, vomiting, diarrhea	Abdominal pain Vaginitis	Rash Jaundice

NURSING CONSIDERATIONS

- PO: peak 45 minutes, duration 6 hours
- IM: peak 3 hours, duration 8–12 hours
- May cause increase in AST, ALT, CPK
- Do not break, crush, or chew capsules
- Rx

• •

SIDE EFFECTS

Nausea, vomiting, diarrhea	Photosensitivity Hepatotoxicity	Angioedema Anemia
Hearing loss	Increased liver	
Dizziness, vertigo	function tests	
Rash	Vaginitis	

NURSING CONSIDERATIONS

- PO: rapid onset, peak 2.5–3.2 hours, duration 24 hours
- IV: rapid onset, peak end of infusion, duration 24 hours
- PO: don't take with antacids; can take with or without food
- Monitor for signs of superinfection (sore throat, fever, fatigue)
- If treated for nongonococcal urethritis or cervicitis, sexual partners also need treatment
- Increases effects of oral anticoagulants
- Rx

CLARITHROMYCIN
(kla-<u>rith</u>-row-my-sin)

(Biaxin, Biaxin XL)

Purpose: treatment of respiratory, skin, and sinus infections

. . . .

ERYTHROMYCIN
(eh-rith-roe-<u>my</u>-sin)

(Ery-Tab, Erythrocin)

Purpose: treatment of mild to moderate respiratory and skin infections, chlamydia, and syphilis

SIDE EFFECTS

Nausea, vomiting, diarrhea

Headache

Taste abnormalities

Ventricular dysrhythmias

Vaginitis

Leukopenia

Rash

NURSING CONSIDERATIONS

- Treatment may be 7–14 days depending on organism and extent of infection
- Medication should be taken with food
- Be aware of possible increase in theophylline, carbamazepine, and digoxin levels
- Monitor for signs of superinfection (sore throat, fever, fatigue)
- Rx

• •

SIDE EFFECTS

Abdominal cramps

Pain at injection site

Nausea, vomiting, diarrhea

Rash

Anaphylaxis

Vaginitis

Dysrhythmias

Hepatotoxicity

NURSING CONSIDERATIONS

- PO: give 1 hour before or 2 hours after meals
- PO: give with full glass of water; avoid citrus juice
- PO: onset 1 hour, peak up to 4 hours, duration 6–12 hours
- IV: onset rapid, peak end of infusion, duration 6–12 hours
- Take at equal intervals around the clock
- Can be used in patients with compromised renal function
- Monitor for signs of superinfection (sore throat, fever, fatigue)
- Rx

AMOXICILLIN, AMPICILLIN, PENICILLIN
(ah-mox-i-<u>sill</u>-in, am-pi-<u>sill</u>-in, pen-i-<u>sill</u>-in)

(Bicillin, Omnipen, Wycillin)

Purpose: treatment of respiratory, skin, gastrointestinal, and urinary infections and of otitis media and gonorrhea

• •

TRIMETHOPRIM/SULFAMETHOXAZOLE
(trye-<u>meth</u>-a-prim sul-fa-meth-<u>ox</u>-a-zole)

(Bactrim, Septra)

Purpose: treatment of urinary tract infections, otitis media, chronic prostatitis, shigellosis, chancroid, and traveler's diarrhea

SIDE EFFECTS

Allergic reactions: fever, difficulty breathing, skin rash

Renal, hepatic, hematologic abnormalities

Nausea, vomiting, diarrhea

Urticaria, rash

Bone marrow suppression

NURSING CONSIDERATIONS

- Take careful history of penicillin reaction; observe for 20 minutes post IM injection
- PO for penicillin and ampicillin: take 1 hour ac or 2 hours pc to reduce gastric acid destruction of drug; not true for amoxicillin
- Take equally divided doses around the clock
- Continue medication for entire time prescribed, even if symptoms resolve
- Check for hypersensitivity to other drugs, especially cephalosporins
- Rx

• •

SIDE EFFECTS

Hypersensitivity reaction

Blood dyscrasias

Photosensitivity

Nausea, vomiting, anorexia

Stomatitis, abdominal pain

Headache, fatigue

Bone marrow suppression

Increased BUN/creatinine

NURSING CONSIDERATIONS

- PO: with full glass water; if upset stomach occurs, take with food
- PO: take at equal intervals around the clock
- IV: infuse slowly over 60–90 minutes; flush lines at end of infusion to remove residue
- Monitor for hypersensitivity reaction; stop med at first sign of skin rash
- Never administer IM, rapidly IV, or by bolus injection
- Encourage fluids to 8–10 glasses/day
- Rx

DOXYCYCLINE HYCLATE
(dox-i-<u>sye</u>-kleen <u>hye</u>-klate)

(Vibramycin, Vibra-Tabs)

Purpose: treatment of syphilis, gonorrhea, chlamydia, chronic periodontitis, acne, and anthrax; prophylaxis of malaria

• •

MINOCYCLINE HCL
(mi-noe-<u>sye</u>-kleen)

(Minocin)

Purpose: treatment of syphilis, gonorrhea, chlamydia, periodontitis, acne, bronchitis, and meningitis

SIDE EFFECTS

Photosensitivity

GI upset, diarrhea

Renal, hepatic, hematologic
abnormalities

Dental discoloration of
deciduous (baby) teeth

Rash

NURSING CONSIDERATIONS

- Peak 1.5–4 hours
- If GI symptoms occur, administer with food EXCEPT milk
  products or other foods high in calcium (interferes with
  absorption)
- Take with full glass of water; do NOT take within 1 hour of
  bedtime or reclining
- Avoid during tooth and early development periods (4th month
  prenatal to 8 years of age)
- Increases effects of anticoagulants
- Rx

• •

SIDE EFFECTS

Photosensitivity

GI upset, diarrhea

Renal, hepatic, hematologic
abnormalities

Dental discoloration of
deciduous (baby) teeth

Dizziness

Hepatotoxicity

Urticaria, rash

NURSING CONSIDERATIONS

- Peak 2–3 hours
- If GI symptoms occur, administer with food EXCEPT milk
  products or other foods high in calcium (interferes with
  absorption)
- Take with full glass of water; do NOT take within 1 hour of
  bedtime
- Avoid during tooth and early development periods (4th month
  prenatal to 8 years of age)
- Rx

HYDROCORTISONE
(hye-dro-<u>kor</u>-ti-sone)

(Cortef, Solu-Cortef)

Purpose: treatment of severe inflammation, adrenal insufficiency, ulcerative colitis, collagen disorder, asthma, lupus, and COPD

• •

METHYLPREDNISOLONE
(meth-ill-pred-<u>niss</u>-oh-lone)

(Medrol)

Purpose: treatment of severe inflammation, shock, adrenal insufficiency, collagen disorders; management of acute spinal cord injury and multiple sclerosis

SIDE EFFECTS

Depression
Flushing, sweating
Hypertension
Nausea, diarrhea

Hyperglycemia
Mood changes, euphoria
Blurred vision
Thrombocytopenia

NURSING CONSIDERATIONS

- Med masks signs of infection, so check for elevated temperature, WBC count
- PO: take with food or milk
- IM: give deep into gluteal muscle, avoid deltoid, rotate sites, avoid subQ (may damage tissue)
- Rectal: for colitis, retain med for 60 minutes, onset 3–5 days
- Wear medical information tag
- Do not mix with other medicines
- Rx

• •

SIDE EFFECTS

GI hemorrhage
Hypertension
  and circulatory
  problems

Poor wound
  healing
Hyperglycemia
Mood changes

Thrombocytopenia
Increased IOP
Diarrhea, nausea,
  distention

NURSING CONSIDERATIONS

- PO: take with food or milk
- PO: peak 1–2 hours, duration 1.5 days
- IM: give deep into gluteal muscle, avoid deltoid, rotate sites, avoid subQ (may damage tissue)
- IM: peak 4–8 days, duration 1–4 weeks
- Eat foods high in protein, calcium, vitamin D, and potassium
- Contact provider if anorexia, difficulty breathing, weakness, dizziness; symptoms may appear during periods of stress or trauma
- Contact provider if black/tarry stools, slow wound healing, blurred vision, bruising/bleeding, weight gain, emotional changes
- Wear medical information tag
- Monitor patient weight, blood sugars, and potassium
- Rx

PREDNISOLONE
(pred-<u>niss</u>-oh-lone)

(Delta-Cortef, Flo-Pred, Prelone)

Purpose: treatment of severe inflammation, immunosuppression, neoplasms, and asthma

• •

PREDNISONE
(<u>pred</u>-ni-sone)

(Deltasone, Meticorten)

Purpose: treatment of severe inflammation, immunosuppression, neoplasms, multiple sclerosis, collagen disorders, dermatological disorders, pulmonary fibrosis, and asthma

SIDE EFFECTS

Depression

Hypertension, circulatory problems

Nausea, diarrhea

Abdominal distention

Increased IOP

GI hemorrhage

Tendon rupture

Poor wound healing

Hyperglycemia

NURSING CONSIDERATIONS

- PO: take with food or milk
- PO: peak 1–2 hours, duration 3–36 hours
- IM: give deep into gluteal muscle, avoid deltoid, rotate sites, avoid subQ (may damage tissue)
- IM: peak 1 hour, duration 4 weeks
- Eat food high in protein, calcium, vitamin D, and potassium
- Contact provider if anorexia, difficulty breathing, weakness, dizziness; symptoms may appear during periods of stress or trauma
- Contact provider if black/tarry stools, slow wound healing, blurred vision, bruising/bleeding, weight gain, emotional changes
- Wear medical information tag
- Monitor potassium, glucose, and weight
- Rx

• •

SIDE EFFECTS

GI hemorrhage

Hypertension, circulatory problems

Depression

Nausea, diarrhea

Abdominal distention

Hyperglycemia

Mood changes

Increased IOP

NURSING CONSIDERATIONS

- PO: take with food or milk, antacids
- PO: peak 1–2 hours, duration 24–36 hours
- Eat food high in protein, calcium, vitamin D, and potassium
- Contact provider if anorexia, difficulty breathing, weakness, dizziness; symptoms may appear during periods of stress or trauma
- Contact provider if black/tarry stools, slow wound healing, blurred vision, bruising/bleeding, weight gain, emotional changes
- Excessive consumption of licorice can increase risk of hypokalemia
- Wear medical information tag
- Rx

MELOXICAM
(ma-<u>locks</u>-uh-kam)

(Mobic)

Purpose: treatment of pain or inflammation caused by arthritis

• •

Antineoplastics
Antineoplastics

CISPLATIN
(sis-<u>plat</u>-in)

(Platinol)

Purpose: treatment of advanced bladder cancer, adjunct therapy in metastatic testicular and ovarian cancer

SIDE EFFECTS

Dizziness
GI upset
Nausea, vomiting

URI
Flulike symptoms

NURSING CONSIDERATIONS

- Take without regard to meals
- Rx

. . . .

SIDE EFFECTS

Seizures
Peripheral
  neuropathy
Cardiac
  abnormalities
Ototoxicity
Blurred vision

Stomatitis
Nausea, vomiting
Renal tubular
  damage
Thrombocytopenia,
  leukopenia
Sterility

Alopecia
Hypomagnesemia
Hypocalcemia
Hypokalemia
Hypophosphatemia
Fibrosis

NURSING CONSIDERATIONS

- Use cytotoxic handling procedures
- Give antiemetic 30–60 minutes before treatment
- Monitor temperature every 4 hours
- Increase fluid intake to 2–3 L/day
- Rinse mouth 3–4 times/day for stomatitis
- Avoid vaccinations during therapy
- Rx

CYCLOPHOSPHAMIDE
(sye-kloe-<u>foss</u>-fuh-mide)

(Cytoxan)

Purpose: treatment of cancer

• •

METHOTREXATE
(meth-oh-<u>trex</u>-ate)

(Trexall)

Purpose: treatment of cancer, psoriasis, rheumatoid arthritis, and mycosis fungoides

SIDE EFFECTS

Headache, dizziness
Cardiotoxicity
SIADH
Stomatitis
Nausea, vomiting

Hepatotoxicity
Hemorrhagic crisis
Renal tubular
  necrosis
Sterility

Leukopenia
Alopecia
Hyperuricemia
Pulmonary fibrosis

NURSING CONSIDERATIONS

- Use cytotoxic handling procedures
- Avoid evening dosing
- Give antiemetic 30–60 minutes before treatment
- PO: take on an empty stomach
- Monitor temperature every 4 hours
- Increase fluid intake to 2–3 L/day
- Rinse mouth 3–4 times/day for stomatitis
- Avoid aspirin, ibuprofen
- Avoid vaccinations during therapy
- Rx

• •

SIDE EFFECTS

Nausea, vomiting,
  diarrhea
Anorexia

Alopecia, rash
Ulcerative stomatitis
Dizziness, headache

Renal abnormalities
Hepatotoxicity
Thrombocytopenia

NURSING CONSIDERATIONS

- PO, IM, IV: onset 4–7 days, peak 7–14 days, duration 21 days
- Avoid crowds and people with known infections
- Do not take with ASA or other NSAIDs, which may cause GI bleeding
- Monitor for pulmonary toxicity, which may manifest early as a dry, nonproductive cough
- Do not take with proton pump inhibitors
- Increase fluid intake to 10–12 glasses/day
- Rx

TAMOXiFEN
(ta-<u>mox</u>-i-fen)

Purpose: management of advanced breast cancer not responsive to other therapy in estrogen-receptor-positive patients

• •

Cardiovascular Medications
ACE Inhibitors

BENAZEPRIL HCL
(ben-<u>ay</u>-ze-pril)

(Lotensin)

Purpose: treatment of hypertension

SIDE EFFECTS

Nausea, vomiting
Hot flashes, headache
Rash

Vaginal discharge
Vision abnormalities
Irregular menses
Fluid retention

Depression, mood disturbances
Chest pain

NURSING CONSIDERATIONS

- Peak 4–7 hours
- To decrease GI upset, take after antacid, after evening meal, before bedtime, or take antiemetic 30–60 minutes ahead
- Vaginal bleeding, pruritus, hot flashes are reversible after stopping med
- Contact provider if decreased visual acuity, which may be irreversible
- Tumor flare (increase in tumor size and increased bone pain) may occur, but will decrease rapidly; may take analgesics for pain
- Rx

• •

SIDE EFFECTS

Angioedema
Cough
Headache
Dizziness

Fatigue
Hyperkalemia
Nausea, vomiting, constipation

Hepatotoxicity
Increased renal lab values

NURSING CONSIDERATIONS

- Often used in combination with thiazide diuretics
- Avoid salt substitutes containing potassium because of potassium-sparing effect
- Avoid nonprescription cough medications unless provider directed
- Rx

CAPTOPRIL
(<u>kap</u>-toe-pril)

(Capoten)

Purpose: treatment of hypertension, CHF, left ventricular dysfunction after MI, and diabetic nephropathy

. . . .

ENALAPRIL
(e-<u>nal</u>-a-pril)

(Vasotec)

Purpose: treatment of hypertension, CHF, and left ventricular dysfunction

SIDE EFFECTS

Bronchospasm, dyspnea, cough
Orthostatic hypotension

Dizziness
Loss of taste
Nephrotic syndrome

Bone marrow suppression
Hyperkalemia

NURSING CONSIDERATIONS

- Contact provider if fever, skin rash, sore throat, mouth sores, swelling of hands or feet, fast or irregular heartbeat, chest pain, or cough
- Take on empty stomach 1 hour before meals or 2 hours after; tablets may be crushed and mixed with juice or soft food for ease of swallowing
- Avoid changing positions (sitting/standing/lying) rapidly, esp. during the first few days before body adjusts to med
- Do not use OTC (cough, cold, or allergy) meds unless directed by provider
- Avoid potassium supplements, potassium salt substitute, and potassium-sparing diuretics
- Rx

• •

SIDE EFFECTS

Headache
Dizziness, hypotension
Tachycardia, dysrhythmias

Tinnitus
Hyperkalemia
Angioedema
Persistent cough
Insomnia

Bone marrow suppression
Hepatotoxity
Renal failure

NURSING CONSIDERATIONS

- Contact provider if fever, skin rash, sore throat, mouth sores, swelling of hands or feet, fast or irregular heartbeat, chest pain, or cough
- Avoid changing positions (sitting/standing/lying) rapidly, esp. during the first few days before body adjusts to med
- Do not use OTC (cough, cold, or allergy) meds unless directed by provider
- Avoid potassium supplements, potassium salt substitutes, and potassium-sparing diuretics
- May be crushed; give without regard to food
- Rx

LISINOPRIL
(lye-<u>sin</u>-oh-pril)

(Prinivil, Zestril)

Purpose: treatment of mild to moderate hypertension, adjunctive therapy for systolic CHF and acute MI

• •

RAMIPRIL
(<u>ram</u>-ih-pril)

(Altace)

Purpose: treatment of hypertension and CHF following MI; prophylactic risk reduction of MI, stroke, and death from cardiovascular disorders

SIDE EFFECTS

Headache, fatigue

Dizziness, vertigo

Nausea, vomiting, diarrhea

Hypotension

Tachycardia

Cough

Renal insufficiency

Hepatic failure

Hyperkalemia

NURSING CONSIDERATIONS

- Avoid changing positions (lying/sitting/standing) rapidly
- May take without regard to food
- Avoid potassium supplements, potassium salt substitutes, and potassium-sparing diuretics
- Rx

• •

SIDE EFFECTS

Headache, fatigue

Hypotension

Dizziness, vertigo

Nausea, vomiting, diarrhea

Cough

Hyperkalemia

Altered renal and hepatic function tests

Decreased Hgb and Hct

NURSING CONSIDERATIONS

- Can mix capsule contents with water, juice, or applesauce to aid swallowing
- Avoid changing positions (lying/sitting/standing) rapidly
- Contact provider if persistent dry, nonproductive cough; increased SOB; edema; or unusual bruising or bleeding
- Avoid potassium supplements, potassium salt substitutes, and potassium-sparing diuretics
- Rx

DOXAZOSIN MESYLATE
(dox-<u>ay</u>-zoe-sin <u>mes</u>-i-late)

(Cardura)

Purpose: treatment of hypertension and benign prostatic hyperplasia

• •

PRAZOSIN HCL
(<u>pray</u>-zoh-sin)

(Minipress)

Purpose: treatment of hypertension

SIDE EFFECTS

Dizziness, vertigo
Orthostatic hypotension
Headache
Tinnitus

Fatigue, malaise
Priapism (rare)
Nausea, vomiting, diarrhea

NURSING CONSIDERATIONS

- Avoid changing positions (lying/sitting/standing) rapidly
- Can have first-dose syncope, maintain recumbent for 90 minutes
- Use caution in potentially hazardous activities until stabilized
- Rx

• •

SIDE EFFECTS

Dizziness, drowsiness
Nausea, vomiting, diarrhea
Headache, vertigo
Palpitations

Syncope
Blurred vision
Nasal congestion

NURSING CONSIDERATIONS

- Onset 2 hours, peak 1–3 hours, duration 6–12 hours
- Can have first-dose syncope; take the first dose (and any increment) at bedtime, do not drive for 24 hours
- Full therapeutic effects may require 4–6 weeks of therapy
- Food may delay absorption
- Avoid changing positions (lying/sitting/standing) rapidly
- Check with provider before using OTC cold, cough, and allergy meds
- Rx

TERAZOSIN HCL
(ter-<u>ay</u>-zoh-sin)

(Hytrin)

Purpose: treatment of hypertension and benign prostatic hyperplasia

• •

LOSARTAN
(loe-<u>sar</u>-tan)

(Cozaar)

Purpose: treatment of hypertension

SIDE EFFECTS

Dizziness, weakness
Headache, drowsiness
Nausea

Syncope
Blurred vision
Nasal congestion

NURSING CONSIDERATIONS

- Avoid changing positions (lying/sitting/standing) rapidly
- Can have first-dose syncope, take the first dose (and any increment) at bedtime; do not drive or operate machinery for 4 hours
- Check with provider before using OTC cold, cough, and allergy meds
- Rx

● ●

SIDE EFFECTS

Dizziness, confusion	Diarrhea, anorexia	Photosensitivity
Insomnia	Dyspepsia	Alopecia, rash
Headache	Impotence	Hyperkalemia
Dysrhythmias, MI	Renal failure	Hypoglycemia
Blurred vision	Thrombocytopenia	URI

NURSING CONSIDERATIONS

- Avoid hazardous activities until reaction is known
- Avoid grapefruit juice, alcohol, salt substitutes, OTC products
- Take without regard to meals
- Rx

VALSARTAN
(val-<u>sar</u>-tan)

(Diovan)

Purpose: treatment of hypertension, treatment of heart failure in patients who cannot take ACE inhibitors, reduction of cardiovascular mortality post-MI in stable patients with left ventricular dysfunction/failure

• •

VALSARTAN HYDROCHLOROTHIAZIDE
(val-<u>sar</u>-tan hye-droe-klor-oh-<u>thye</u>-a-zide)

(Diovan HCT)

Purpose: treatment of hypertension, treatment of heart failure in patients who cannot take ACE inhibitors

SIDE EFFECTS

Headache

Dizziness, vertigo

Abdominal pain

Nausea, vomiting,
  diarrhea

Hypotension

Cough

Dysrhythmias

Hepatotoxicity

Nephrotoxicity

Hyperkalemia

Angioedema

NURSING CONSIDERATIONS

- Take once daily for high blood pressure, twice daily for CHF
- Avoid potassium supplements and salt substitutes containing potassium
- Give on an empty stomach
- Rx

• •

SIDE EFFECTS

Headache

Dizziness, vertigo

Nausea, vomiting,
  diarrhea

Hypotension

Cough

Blurred vision

Photosensitivity

Agranulocytosis

Nephrotoxicity

Hepatotoxicity

Hyperglycemia

Hypokalemia/
  hyperkalemia

NURSING CONSIDERATIONS

- Take once daily for high blood pressure, twice daily for CHF
- Avoid potassium supplements and salt substitutes containing potassium
- NSAIDs may reduce the effect of diuretic
- May cause exacerbation of SLE
- Rx

ISOSORBIDE DINITRATE

(eye-soe-<u>sor</u>-bide)

(Isordil)

Purpose: treatment and prevention of chronic stable angina

• •

ISOSORBIDE MONONITRATE

(eye-soe-<u>sor</u>-bide)

(Ismo)

Purpose: treatment and prevention of chronic stable angina

SIDE EFFECTS

Dizziness, orthostatic
hypotension
Vascular headache, flushing

Drowsiness
Nausea, vomiting
Lightheadedness

NURSING CONSIDERATIONS

- PO: 1 hour before food or 2 hours after meals for maximum absorption, but taking with food may reduce or eliminate headache
- Chewable tablet: chew well, hold in mouth for 2 minutes before swallowing
- SL: dissolve under tongue; do not eat, drink, talk, or smoke during use; go to ED if pain not relieved in 15 minutes
- Avoid changing positions (lying/sitting/standing) rapidly
- Use caution in potentially hazardous activities until stabilized
- Avoid alcohol, smoking, strenuous exercise in hot environment
- Wear medical information tag
- Rx

• •

SIDE EFFECTS

Dizziness, postural
hypotension

Vascular headache,
flushing

Drowsiness
Nausea, vomiting

NURSING CONSIDERATIONS

- PO: 1 hour before food or 2 hours after meals for maximum absorption, but taking with food may reduce or eliminate headache
- Chewable tablet: chew well, hold in mouth for 2 minutes before swallowing
- SL: dissolve under tongue; do not eat, drink, talk, or smoke during use; go to ED if pain not relieved in 15 minutes
- Avoid changing positions (lying/sitting/standing) rapidly
- Use caution in potentially hazardous activities until stabilized
- Avoid alcohol, smoking, strenuous exercise in hot environment
- Wear medical information tag
- Rx

NITROGLYCERIN
(nye-troe-<u>gli</u>-ser-in)

(Nitro-Par, Transderm-Nitro/Nitrostat)

Purpose: treatment of chronic stable angina; prophylaxis of angina pain, CHF, and acute MI; controlled hypotension for surgical procedures

• •

AMIODARONE HCL
(am-ee-<u>oh</u>-da-rone)

(Cordarone, Pacerone)

Purpose: management of ventricular arrhythmias not controlled by first-line agents

SIDE EFFECTS

Postural hypotension
Nausea, vomiting
Headache, flushing, dizziness

NURSING CONSIDERATIONS

- Sustained-release: take every 6–12 hours on an empty stomach; onset 20–45 minutes, duration 3–8 hours
- SL: patient sitting/lying should let tablet dissolve under tongue and not swallow saliva; onset 1–3 minutes, duration 30 minutes
- Spray: hold canister vertically, spray on tongue, close mouth immediately, do not inhale spray; onset 2 minutes, duration 30–60 minutes
- IV: use infusion pump and special non-PVC tubing; onset 1–2 minutes, duration 3–5 minutes
- Ointment: spread on skin in thin uniform layer; onset 30–60 minutes, duration 2–12 hours
- Transdermal: apply to clean hairless area; rotate sites; onset 30–60 minutes, duration 12–24 hours
- Go to ED if pain not relieved with 3 tablets in 15 minutes
- Wear medical information tag
- Rx

• •

SIDE EFFECTS

Dizziness, fatigue, malaise
Anorexia, constipation
Nausea, vomiting
Bradycardia, hypotension

Corneal microdeposits
Photosensitivity
Hypo/ hyperthyroidism
Muscle weakness
Cardiac arrest

Peripheral neuropathy
Hepatotoxicity
Rash
Neurotoxicity

NURSING CONSIDERATIONS

- IV: continuous cardiac monitoring
- Assess for signs of pulmonary toxicity: rales/crackles, decreased breath sounds, pleuritic friction rub, fatigue, dyspnea, cough, pleuritic pain, fever
- Side effects may not appear until several days, weeks, or years and may persist for several months after stopping med
- Teach patient to check radial pulse
- May increase ALT, AST
- Rx

FLECAINIDE
(fleh-<u>kay</u>-nide)

(Tambocor)

Purpose: management of life-threatening ventricular dysrhythmias, sustained ventricular tachycardia, and atrial flutter/fibrillation

• •

LIDOCAINE HCL
(<u>lye</u>-doe-kane)

(Xylocaine)

Purpose: management of ventricular tachycardia and ventricular dysrhythmias during cardiac surgery

SIDE EFFECTS

Headache
Dizziness, irritability
Suppression
Tremors
Hypotension,
  bradycardia

CHF
Tachycardia
Blurred vision
Tinnitus
Nausea, vomiting,
  constipation

Change in taste
Impotence
Urinary retention
Leukopenia
Respiratory
  depression

NURSING CONSIDERATIONS

- Take with meals to minimize GI upset
- May adjust dose every 4 days
- Reduce dosage as soon as dysrhythmia is controlled
- Avoid changing positions rapidly
- Do not skip or double doses; if dose missed, take as soon as possible within 6 hours of next dose
- Wear medical identification tag
- Rx

• •

SIDE EFFECTS

Hypotension, tremors
Blurred vision
Tinnitus
Respiratory depression/arrest
Confusion

Drowsiness, dizziness
Seizures
Bradycardia
Nausea, vomiting, anorexia
Rash, petechiae

NURSING CONSIDERATIONS

- Give oxygen; have resuscitation equipment available
- IV: use infusion pump; patient on cardiac monitor
- Rx

PROCAINAMIDE
(proe-<u>kane</u>-a-mide)

Purpose: management of life-threatening ventricular dysrhythmias

• •

QUINIDINE
(<u>kwin</u>-i-deen)

Purpose: management of atrial or ventricular arrhythmias and malaria

SIDE EFFECTS

Hypotension
Nausea, vomiting
Fever, rash
Dizziness

Bone marrow suppression
SLE syndrome
Confusion, restlessness
Angioedema

NURSING CONSIDERATIONS

- IV: use infusion pump; monitor BP every 5–15 minutes; on cardiac monitor; keep patient recumbent
- IV: monitor CBC, blood levels, I&O, daily weight
- May increase alkaline phosphatase, bilirium, AST, ALT
- Rx

• •

SIDE EFFECTS

Anemia
Hypotension, bradycardia
Nausea, vomiting, diarrhea
Headache, dizziness
Heart block

Tinnitus
Vision changes
Respiratory depression
Hepatotoxicity
Thrombocytopenia

NURSING CONSIDERATIONS

- May increase toxicity for digitalis
- Monitor EKG, BP, and pulse
- Avoid changing positions (lying/sitting/standing) rapidly
- Avoid use with alcohol, caffeine, smoking
- Wear medical information tag
- Rx

SOTALOL
(<u>soe</u>-ta-lole)

(Betapace)

Purpose: management of life-threatening ventricular arrhythmias

• •

BISOPROLOL
(bis-<u>oh</u>-pro-lole)

(Zebeta)

Purpose: treatment of mild to moderate hypertension

SIDE EFFECTS

Fatigue
Weakness
Dizziness,
  drowsiness
Bradycardia

Life-threatening
  ventricular
  arrhythmias
Dyspnea,
  bronchospasms

Nausea, vomiting,
  diarrhea
Hyperglycemia
Impotence
Visual changes

NURSING CONSIDERATIONS

- Teach patient to check radial pulse; if less than 50, hold med and contact provider
- PO: give 1 hour before or 1 hour after meals
- Change positions (sitting/standing/lying) slowly
- Avoid activities that require alertness until drug response known
- Contact provider if slow pulse, difficulty breathing, wheezing, cold hands and feet, dizziness, confusion, depression, rash, fever, sore throat, unusual bleeding or bruising
- Milk products may decrease absorption
- Wear medical information tag
- Avoid alcohol, smoking, and sodium intake
- Rx

• •

SIDE EFFECTS

GI upset
Dizziness, vertigo
Headache, fatigue
Bronchospasms, dyspnea

Postural hypotension
Impotence
Increased AST/ALT

NURSING CONSIDERATIONS

- Peak: 2–4 hours
- Therapeutic response in 1–2 weeks
- Do not stop med abruptly; may precipitate angina
- Do not use OTC meds with stimulants, such as nasal decongestants or cold meds, unless directed
- Avoid alcohol, smoking, sodium intake
- Contact provider if signs of CHF: difficulty breathing, night cough, swelling of extremities
- Teach patient to check radial pulse
- Rx

CLONIDINE PATCH
(<u>kloe</u>-ni-deen)

(Catapres, Catapres TTS oral tablets)

Purpose: treatment of hypertension, severe pain in cancer patients, and ADHD

• •

HYDRALAZINE HCL
(hye-<u>dral</u>-a-zeen)

Purpose: treatment of essential hypertension and hypertensive emergency

SIDE EFFECTS

Drowsiness, sedation

Severe rebound hypertension

Dry mouth and eyes

Hyperglycemia

Nausea, vomiting, constipation

Orthostatic hypotension

Impotence

Taste change

Dizziness

Headache

Rash

NURSING CONSIDERATIONS

- Avoid changing positions (lying/sitting/standing) rapidly
- Avoid use with alcohol, CNS depressants or OTC meds with stimulants
- Avoid high-sodium foods (canned soups, lunch meats, cheese)
- Avoid alcohol, smoking, strenuous exercise in hot environment
- Apply patch to nonhairy area (upper outer arm, anterior chest), rotate sites, do not apply to scarred or irritated area
- Wear medical information tag
- Rx

• •

SIDE EFFECTS

Headache

Palpitations, tachycardia, angina

Edema

Lupus erythematosus-like syndrome

Anorexia

Dizziness

Anxiety

Rash

Nausea, vomiting, diarrhea

Hepatotoxicity

Leukopenia

Orthostatic hypotension

NURSING CONSIDERATIONS

- Avoid changing positions (lying/sitting/standing) rapidly
- Contact provider if chest pain, severe fatigue, fever, muscle, or joint pain
- Do not confuse with hydroxyzine
- Rx

HYDROCHLOROTHIAZIDE/ LISINOPRIL
(hye-droe-klor-oh-<u>thye</u>-a-zide/ lye-<u>sin</u>-oh-pril)

(Prinzide, Zestoretic)

Purpose: treatment of essential hypertension

• •

Cardiovascular Medications
Antilipemic Agents

ATORVASTATIN CALCIUM
(a-<u>tor</u>-va-stat-in)

(Lipitor)

Purpose: reduction of cholesterol levels

SIDE EFFECTS

Headache

Dizziness, vertigo

Nausea, vomiting,
  diarrhea

Hypotension

Tachycardia

Cough

Muscle cramps

Angioedema

Hyperkalemia

Hepatic failure

Renal insufficiency

NURSING CONSIDERATIONS

- Avoid changing positions (lying/sitting/standing) rapidly
- May take without regard to food
- Avoid potassium supplements, potassium salt substitutes, and potassium-sparing diuretics
- Rx

• •

SIDE EFFECTS

Constipation

Abdominal pain

Nausea, diarrhea

Arthralgia

Impotence

Headache, insomnia

Increased liver
  enzymes

Lens opacities

NURSING CONSIDERATIONS

- Peak 1–2 hours
- Take without regard to food
- Avoid grapefruit products
- Contact provider immediately if unexplained muscle pain, tenderness, or weakness; in rare cases, can cause breakdown of skeletal muscle tissue, leading to kidney failure
- Rx

EZETIMIBE
(e-<u>zet</u>-i-mibe)

(Zetia)

Purpose: reduction of cholesterol levels

• •

FENOFIBRATE
(fen-oh-<u>fye</u>-brate)

(Tricor)

Purpose: reduction of cholesterol levels

SIDE EFFECTS

Diarrhea, abdominal pain
Joint pain, arthralgia

Fatigue, dizziness
URI, sinusitis

NURSING CONSIDERATIONS

- Ezetimibe is not a statin; can be used with a statin or alone; works by removing cholesterol from the small intestine (statins work in the liver)
- Contact provider immediately if unexplained muscle pain, tenderness, or weakness; in rare cases, can cause breakdown of skeletal muscle tissue, leading to kidney failure
- Take without regard to meals
- Peak 4–12 hours
- Rx

• •

SIDE EFFECTS

Fatigue, weakness
Insomnia
Depression
Hypo/hypertension
Nausea, vomiting, dyspepsia

Increased liver enzymes
Pancreatitis
Dysuria
Leukopenia
Photosensitivity

Rash
Weight gain
Myalgia
Cough

NURSING CONSIDERATIONS

- Contact provider if unexplained muscle pain, tenderness, or weakness; in rare cases can cause breakdown of skeletal muscle tissue, leading to kidney failure
- Avoid changing positions rapidly
- Rx

FLUVASTATIN
(<u>floo</u>-va-stat-in)

(Lescol)

Purpose: reduction of cholesterol levels, secondary prevention of coronary events in patients with CAD

• •

GEMFIBROZIL
(jem-<u>fye</u>-bruh-zill)

(Lopid)

Purpose: reduction of cholesterol levels

SIDE EFFECTS

Confusion
Urinary pain
Headache, dizziness
Hepatotoxicity
Photosensitivity

Abdominal pain, constipation
Nausea, diarrhea
Arthralgia
Thrombocytopenia

NURSING CONSIDERATIONS

- Contact provider immediately if unexplained muscle pain, tenderness, or weakness; in rare cases, can cause breakdown of skeletal muscle tissue, leading to kidney failure
- Take without regard to meals
- Peak response 3–4 weeks
- Rx

● ●

SIDE EFFECTS

Fatigue, vertigo
Headache
Dyspepsia
Nausea, vomiting, diarrhea
Abdominal pain

Leukopenia
Rash, urticaria
Taste perversion
Myopathy
Angioedema

NURSING CONSIDERATIONS

- Administer 30 minutes before a.m. and p.m. meals
- Monitor blood glucose, renal/hepatic studies in long-term therapy
- Avoid alcohol, high-fat diet, smoking, sedentary lifestyle
- Rx

LOVASTATIN
(<u>loh</u>-vah-stat-in)

(Mevacor)

Purpose: reduction of cholesterol levels

· ·

NIACIN (NICOTINIC ACID)
(<u>nye</u>-a-sin)

(Niacor for immediate release, Niaspan for sustained release, Slo-Niacin, vitamin B)

Purpose: treatment of pellagra, hyperlipidemia, and peripheral vascular disease

SIDE EFFECTS

Flatus, constipation
Abdominal pain, nausea,
diarrhea, GI upset
Heartburn

Muscle cramps
Dizziness
Headache
Tremor
Blurred vision

Rash, pruritus
Photosensitivity
Increased liver function tests

NURSING CONSIDERATIONS

- Onset 2 weeks, peak 4–6 weeks, duration 6 weeks
- Take with food, absorption is reduced by 30% on an empty stomach
- Contact provider if unexplained muscle pain, tenderness, or weakness; in rare cases can cause breakdown of skeletal muscle tissue leading to kidney failure
- Avoid grapefruit products
- Rx

• •

SIDE EFFECTS

Headache
Nausea, vomiting
Postural hypotension

Myopathy
Flushing
Pruritus

Abnormalities of liver function tests
Hyperglycemia

NURSING CONSIDERATIONS

- Take with meals to reduce GI upset, can add 325 mg ASA 30 minutes before dose to reduce flushing
- Flushing will occur several hours after med taken, will decrease over 2 weeks
- Avoid changing positions (sitting/standing/lying) rapidly
- May be used in combination with simvastatin or lovastatin
- OTC, Rx

PRAVASTATIN
(<u>prav</u>-a-stat-in)

(Pravachol)

Purpose: reduction of cholesterol levels and risk of recurrent MI, treatment of atherosclerosis

• •

ROSUVASTATIN CALCIUM
(roe-<u>sue</u>-vuh-stat-in)

(Crestor)

Purpose: reduction of cholesterol levels and progression of atherosclerosis, prophylaxis of cardiovascular disease and stroke

SIDE EFFECTS

Abdominal cramps, flatus
Heartburn
Constipation, diarrhea
Headache, dizziness, fatigue

Lens opacities
Renal failure
Muscle cramps
Hepatic dysfunction

NURSING CONSIDERATIONS

- Take without regard to food
- Contact provider if unexplained muscle pain, tenderness, or weakness; in rare cases can cause breakdown of skeletal muscle tissue leading to kidney failure
- Peak 1–1.5 hours
- Rx

• •

SIDE EFFECTS

Myalgia
Constipation, heartburn
Abdominal pain
Rash, pruritus

Nausea
Thrombocytopenia
Muscle cramps, arthralgia
Headache, dizziness

Kidney failure
Liver dysfunction

NURSING CONSIDERATIONS

- Patient should keep tight control of diet during therapy
- Contact provider if unexplained muscle pain, tenderness, or weakness; in rare cases can cause breakdown of skeletal muscle tissue leading to kidney failure
- Asian patients may require lower dose at initiation of therapy
- Take without regard to meals
- Rx

SIMVASTATIN

(<u>sim</u>-va-stat-in)

(Zocor)

Purpose: reduction of cholesterol, triglyceride, and lipoprotein levels; prophylaxis of MI and stroke

• •

ATENOLOL

(a-<u>ten</u>-oh-lole)

(Tenormin)

Purpose: treatment of mild to moderate hypertension and MI, prophylaxis of angina

SIDE EFFECTS

Liver dysfunction
URI
Headache

Abdominal pain
Constipation
Nausea

Muscle cramps,
 myalgia
Hyperglycemia

NURSING CONSIDERATIONS

- Take without regard to food
- Contact provider if unexplained muscle pain, tenderness, or weakness; in rare cases can cause breakdown of skeletal muscle tissue leading to kidney failure
- Asian patients should not take niacin while taking simvastatin
- May require lower dose at initiation of therapy
- Rx

• •

SIDE EFFECTS

Bradycardia, cold
 extremities
Postural
 hypotension
Bronchospasm in
 overdose

2nd- or 3rd-degree
 heart block
Cold extremities
Insomnia, fatigue
Dizziness
Mental changes

Nausea, diarrhea
Hypoglycemia
Impotence
Thrombocytopenia

NURSING CONSIDERATIONS

- Masks signs of hypoglycemia in diabetics
- Check pulse; if less than 50 beats per minute, hold the med and contact provider
- PO: take before meals, at bedtime
- Do not stop abruptly; taper over 2 weeks
- Limit alcohol, smoking, sodium intake
- Rx

CARVEDILOL
(kar-<u>ved</u>-i-lole)

(Coreg)

Purpose: treatment of hypertension, CHF, LV dysfunction after MI, and cardiomyopathy

• •

METOPROLOL
(meh-<u>toe</u>-proe-lole)

(Toprol XL, the sustained-release form; Lopressor, the immediate-release form)

Purpose: treatment of hypertension, acute MI, angina, heart failure, and cardiomyopathy

SIDE EFFECTS

Dizziness, fatigue
Diarrhea
Postural
  hypotension
Impotence

Hyperglycemia
CHF worsening
Paresthesia
Bradycardia
Peripheral edema

Headache, insomnia
Increased liver
  enzymes
Thrombocytopenia
Bronchospasm

NURSING CONSIDERATIONS

- PO: take with food
- Tablet may be crushed or swallowed whole
- Do not stop abruptly; taper over 1–2 weeks
- Rx

. . . .

SIDE EFFECTS

Bradycardia,
  palpitations
Nausea, vomiting,
  diarrhea
Hypotension,
  dizziness

CHF
Depression
Insomnia
Confusion,
  headache
Impotence

Bronchospasms
Rash, urticaria
Hypoglycemia

NURSING CONSIDERATIONS

- Check pulse; if less than 60 beats per minute, hold med and contact provider
- PO: may be taken with food, take at same time each day
- XL tablet must be swallowed whole
- Do not stop abruptly; taper over 2 weeks; may precipitate angina
- Do not use OTC products (nasal decongestants, cold preparations) unless directed by provider
- May worsen heart failure
- Rx

PROPRANOLOL HCL
(proe-<u>pran</u>-oh-lole)

(Inderal)

Purpose: treatment of stable angina, hypertension, supraventricular dysrhythmias, and acute MI; prophylaxis of migraine

• •

Cardiovascular Medications
Calcium Channel Blockers

AMLODIPINE
(am-<u>loh</u>-di-peen)

(Norvasc)

Purpose: treatment of chronic stable angina, hypertension, and variant angina

SIDE EFFECTS

Weakness, fatigue
Hypotension, dizziness
Impotence
Bronchospasm
Bradycardia
Nausea, vomiting

Depression
Blurred vision
Hyper/hypoglycemia
Dysrhythmias
Thrombocytopenia
Arthralgia

NURSING CONSIDERATIONS

- Check pulse; if less than 50 beats per minute, hold the med and contact provider
- PO: take with full glass of water at the same time each day
- Do not open, chew, or crush extended-release capsule
- Do not stop abruptly; taper over 2 weeks; may precipitate life-threatening dysrhythmias
- Do not use aluminum-containing antacid; may decrease absorption
- Rx

• •

SIDE EFFECTS

Flushing
Headache, fatigue
Nausea, vomiting
Abdominal pain

Somnolence
Peripheral edema
Nocturia
Sexual difficulties

Palpitations, bradycardia
Cough, dyspnea

NURSING CONSIDERATIONS

- May be taken without regard to meals
- Consult provider before taking nonprescription cough remedies
- Check pulse; if less than 50 beats per minute, hold med and contact provider
- Change positions slowly
- Avoid grapefruit juice
- Rx

DILTIAZEM HCL
(dil-<u>tye</u>-a-zem)

(Cardizem, Dilacor, Tiazac, Cardizem CD [once a day])

Purpose: management of angina, vasospasms, hypertension, atrial fibrillation/flutter, and supraventricular tachycardia

• •

FELODIPINE
(fe-<u>loe</u>-di-peen)

Purpose: treatment of essential hypertension

SIDE EFFECTS

Edema
Nausea, constipation
Rash
Photosensitivity
Headache, dizziness

Fatigue, drowsiness
Bradycardia, palpitations
Increased liver enzymes

Renal failure
Nocturia
CHF, dysrhythmias

NURSING CONSIDERATIONS

- Monitor blood pressure during dosage adjustments
- PO: take on an empty stomach with a full glass of water
- Teach patient how to take radial pulse and keep records of pulse rate; if less than 50 beats per minute, hold dose and notify provider
- Avoid hazardous activities until stabilized on drug
- Do not crush, chew, or break
- Do not stop abruptly
- Avoid grapefruit juice
- Rx

• •

SIDE EFFECTS

Dysrhythmia
Headache
Fatigue, dizziness
Edema, CHF
Flushing

Nausea, vomiting, diarrhea
Increased liver function tests
Sexual dysfunction

Nocturia
SOB, wheezing

NURSING CONSIDERATIONS

- Do not adjust dosage at intervals of less than 2 weeks
- PO: take without regard to meals
- Do not open, chew, or crush extended-release capsule
- Do not use OTC products or alcohol unless directed by provider; limit caffeine
- Avoid grapefruit juice
- Contact provider if pulse is less than 50 beats per minute
- Rx

NIFEDIPINE
(nye-<u>fed</u>-i-peen)

(Adalat CC, Procardia XL)

Purpose: treatment of hypertension and angina

• •

VERAPAMIL HCL
(ver-<u>ap</u>-a-mill)

(Calan, Covera)

Purpose: treatment of angina, dysrhythmias, hypertension, supraventricular tachycardia, and atrial flutter/fibrillation

SIDE EFFECTS

Orthostatic hypotension
Gingival hyperplasia
Peripheral edema
Palpitations
Headache, dizziness
Fatigue
Nausea, vomiting
Rash
Blurred vision
Flushing
Dysrhythmias
Sexual difficulties
Cough, fever, chills

NURSING CONSIDERATIONS

- Avoid changing positions (sitting/standing/lying) rapidly
- Take without regard to meals; onset 20 minute, peak 6 hours, duration 6–8 hours
- PO, extended-release capsule: do not open, chew, or crush
- Do not use OTC products or alcohol unless directed by provider; limit caffeine
- Monitor BP when used with beta blockers
- Do not drink grapefruit juice; stop grapefruit juice at least 3 days prior to initiating nifedipine therapy
- Protect med from light and store in dry area
- Rx

• •

SIDE EFFECTS

Edema
Nausea, constipation
Headache
Drowsiness
Fatigue
CHF
Dizziness
Bruising
Dysrhythmias
Impotence
Nocturia
Rash

NURSING CONSIDERATIONS

- PO: take before meals, except sustained-release which is to be taken with food
- Do not open, chew, or crush sustained- or extended-release capsule
- Teach patient how to take radial pulse and keep record of pulse rate
- Avoid hazardous activities until stabilized on drug
- Do not use OTC products or alcohol unless directed by provider; limit caffeine
- Avoid grapefruit juice
- Rx

DIGOXIN
(di-<u>jox</u>-in)

(Lanoxin)

Purpose: treatment of heart failure and atrial fibrillation

• •

BUMETANIDE
(byoo-<u>met</u>-a-nide)

(Bumex, Burinex)

Purpose: treatment of edema in CHF

SIDE EFFECTS

Headache
Fatigue
Bradycardia
Nausea

Atrial tachycardia
  (in children)
Blurred vision
Mental disturbances

Vomiting
Dysrhythmias

NURSING CONSIDERATIONS

- Check pulse; if less than 60 beats per minute (adult) or 90 beats per minute (infant), hold the med and contact provider
- PO: with or without food; may crush tablets and mix with food/fluids
- Do not open, chew, or crush capsule
- Contact provider if loss of appetite, lower stomach pain, diarrhea, weakness, drowsiness, headache, blurred or yellow vision, rash, depression
- Eat a sodium-restricted and potassium-rich (bananas, orange juice) diet to keep potassium level normal
- Avoid OTC meds and herbal meds; many adverse interactions may occur
- Do not stop product abruptly
- Rx

• •

SIDE EFFECTS

Electrolyte
  imbalance
Hypovolemia
Ototoxicity
Hyperglycemia
Hypotension

Chest pain
Rash, pruritus
Muscle weakness
Tinnitus
Headache, dizziness
Nausea, diarrhea

Increased
  cholesterol levels
Hypokalemia
Renal failure
Thrombocytopenia
Polyuria

NURSING CONSIDERATIONS

- PO: diuresis onset 30–60 minutes, peak 1–2 hours, duration 3–6 hours
- IM: diuresis onset 40 minutes, peak 1–2 hours, duration 4–6 hours
- IV: diuresis onset 5 minutes, peak 15–30 minutes, duration 3–6 hours
- Weigh daily
- Do not take at bedtime to prevent nocturia
- Encourage potassium-containing foods
- Monitor BUN, CBC, calcium, and uric acid
- Rx

FUROSEMIDE
(fur-<u>oh</u>-se-mide)

(Lasix)

Purpose: treatment of pulmonary edema, edema in CHF and other conditions, and hypertension

• •

CLOPIDOGREL
(klo-<u>pid</u>-oh-grel)

(Plavix)

Purpose: risk reduction for stroke, MI, peripheral arterial disease in high-risk patients, acute coronary syndrome, TIA, and angina

SIDE EFFECTS

Orthostatic
hypotension
Hypokalemia
Hyperglycemia
Nausea, diarrhea

Polyuria
Rash, pruritus
Muscle spasm
Headache, fatigue
Ototoxicity

Renal failure
Electrolyte
imbalances
Thrombocytopenia
Photosensitivity

NURSING CONSIDERATIONS

- PO: diuresis onset 60 minutes, peak 1–2 hours, duration
  6–8 hours
- IV: diuresis onset 5 minutes, peak 30 minutes, duration 2 hours
- PO: take with food or milk to prevent GI upset, slightly lessened
  absorption, tablets may be crushed
- Take early in the day to prevent nocturia and sleeplessness
- Avoid changing positions (sitting/standing/lying) rapidly
- Do not give IV faster than 4 mg/min; may cause ototoxicity
- Rx

• •

SIDE EFFECTS

GI bleeding
Nausea, vomiting, diarrhea,
  GI discomfort
Depression
Bleeding, including life-
  threatening bleeding
Rash

Headache, dizziness
Edema
Chest pain
Glomerulonephritis
Hepatic failure
URI, bronchospasms
Arthralgia

NURSING CONSIDERATIONS

- Monitor blood studies in long-term therapy
- Report signs of unusual bruising, bleeding; it may take longer to
  stop bleeding
- Discontinue 5 days before elective surgery
- Take without regard to food
- Rx

TICLOPIDINE HCL
(tye-<u>cloe</u>-pi-deen)

Purpose: prevention of stroke in high-risk patients

• •

HYDROCHLOROTHIAZIDE/ TRIAMTERENE
(hye-droe-klor-oh-<u>thye</u>-a-zide/trye-<u>am</u>-ter-een)

(Dyazide, Maxzide)

Purpose: treatment of edema and hypertension

SIDE EFFECTS

Rash
Diarrhea
Bleeding
Decrease in WBCs
Thrombocytopenia
Nausea

GI distress
Purpura, rash
Headache, dizziness
Tinnitus
Hypercholesterolemia

NURSING CONSIDERATIONS

- Monitor blood studies in long-term therapy
- Take with meals or just after to decrease gastric symptoms
- Monitor for signs of cholestasis (jaundice, dark urine, light-colored stools)
- Avoid all OTC products unless approved by provider
- Discontinue 10–14 days before surgery
- Rx

• •

SIDE EFFECTS

Nausea, vomiting, diarrhea
Anemia
Renal stones
Hyperkalemia

Hyperglycemia
Muscle cramps
Dizziness, headache
Photosensitivity

NURSING CONSIDERATIONS

- Diuresis onset 2 hours
- Take with meals or just after to decrease gastric symptoms
- Take early in the day to prevent nocturia and sleeplessness
- Diabetes mellitus may become manifest during thiazide treatment
- May increase BUN and serum creatinine
- Rx

SPIRONOLACTONE
(speer-in-oh-<u>lak</u>-tone)

(Aldactone)

*Purpose: treatment of edema and hypertension and of primary
hyperaldosteronism*

• •

CHLORTHALIDONE
(klor-<u>thal</u>-i-done)

(Thalitone, with atenolol Tenoretic)

Purpose: treatment of edema and hypertension

SIDE EFFECTS

Hyperkalemia

Hyponatremia

Vomiting, diarrhea

Bleeding

Rash, pruritus

Gynecomastia

Headache,
  confusion

Impotence

Agranulocytosis

NURSING CONSIDERATIONS

- Diuresis onset 24–48 hours, peak 48–72 hours
- Take in the morning to avoid interference with sleep
- Take with meals or just after to decrease gastric symptoms
- Avoid food high in potassium: oranges, bananas, salt substitutes, dried apricots, dates
- Weigh daily to determine fluid loss; effect of drug may be decreased if used daily
- Contact provider if cramps, lethargy, menstrual abnormalities, deepening voice, breast enlargement
- Avoid potassium supplements
- Monitor electrolytes
- Rx

• •

SIDE EFFECTS

Aplastic anemia

Orthostatic
  hypotension

Nausea, vomiting,
  anorexia

Urinary frequency

Electrolyte changes

Headache, dizziness

Hyperglycemia

Photosensitivity

Rash

Impotence

Hypokalemia

NURSING CONSIDERATIONS

- Diuresis onset 2 hours, peak 6 hours, duration 24–72 hours
- Take with meals or just after to decrease gastric symptoms
- Take in the morning to avoid interference with sleep
- Weigh daily to determine fluid loss; effect of drug may be decreased if used daily
- Avoid changing positions (sitting/standing/lying) rapidly
- Rx

HYDROCHLOROTHIAZIDE
(hye-droe-klor-oh-<u>thye</u>-a-zide)

(Microzide)

Purpose: treatment of edema and hypertension

• •

INDAPAMIDE
(in-<u>dap</u>-a-mide)

Purpose: treatment of edema and hypertension

SIDE EFFECTS

Hypokalemia

Hyperglycemia

Nausea, vomiting, anorexia

Blurred vision

Fatigue, weakness

Confusion, esp. in elderly

Photosensitivity

Orthostatic hypotension

Electrolyte changes

Renal failure

Aplastic anemia

Rash, urticaria

Erectile dysfunction

NURSING CONSIDERATIONS

- Diuresis onset 2 hours, peak 4 hours, duration 6–12 hours
- Take with meals or just after to decrease gastric symptoms
- Take in morning to avoid interference with sleep
- Hypersensitivity to sulfonamide
- Monitor electrolytes
- Rx

• •

SIDE EFFECTS

Headache, dizziness

Electrolyte changes

Orthostatic hypotension

Muscle cramps

Vision disturbances

Nausea, diarrhea

Rash, pruritus

Increased intraocular pressure

Hyperglycemia

Impotence

NURSING CONSIDERATIONS

- Diuresis onset 1–2 hours, peak 2 hours, duration 36 hours
- Take with meals or just after to decrease gastric symptoms, slightly decreased absorption
- Avoid changing positions (sitting/standing/lying) rapidly
- Take in morning to avoid interference with sleep
- Monitor electrolytes
- Rx

METOLAZONE
(meh-<u>tole</u>-a-zone)

(Zaroxolyn, extended-release product)

Purpose: treatment of edema and hypertension

• •

Dermatologicals
Antifungals, Topical

KETOCONAZOLE
(key-toe-<u>kon</u>-a-zole)

(Nizoral)

Purpose: treatment of fungal infections

SIDE EFFECTS

Dizziness, weakness, fatigue

Nausea, vomiting, anorexia

Rash

Hyperglycemia

Hypokalemia

Photosensitivity

Headache

Aplastic anemia

Impotence

Muscle cramps

NURSING CONSIDERATIONS

- Diuresis onset 1 hour, peak 2 hours, duration 12–24 hours
- Take with meals or just after to decrease gastric symptoms, slightly decreased absorption
- Avoid changing positions (sitting/standing/lying) rapidly
- Take in morning to avoid interference with sleep
- Rx

. . . .

SIDE EFFECTS

Photophobia

Rash

Irritation

NURSING CONSIDERATIONS

- Use as topical cream or shampoo
- May require several weeks or months of therapy
- Do not allow shampoo to get in eyes
- Wash hands before and after use
- Contraindicated in patients with sulfite allergy
- Rx

NYSTATIN
(nye-<u>stat</u>-in)

(Mycostatin)

Purpose: treatment of Candida *infections*

• •

FLUOCINONIDE
(floo-oh-<u>sin</u>-oh-nide)

(Lidex, Vanos)

*Purpose: treatment of inflammation and itching caused by psoriasis,
atopic dermatitis, and other skin conditions*

SIDE EFFECTS

GI distress, hypersensitivity
Irritation (with topical use)

NURSING CONSIDERATIONS

- Discontinue if redness, swelling, irritation occurs
- Encourage good oral, vaginal, skin hygiene
- Do not mix oral suspension with food
- Rx

• •

SIDE EFFECTS

Acne
Epidermal thinning
Burning, dryness of skin
Allergic dermatitis

NURSING CONSIDERATIONS

- Topical glucocorticoid
- Apply only to affected areas; do not get in eyes
- Leave site uncovered or lightly covered
- Occlusive dressing is not recommended, systemic absorption may occur
- Do not use on weeping, denuded, or infected areas
- Avoid sunlight on affected areas
- Rx

TRIAMCINOLONE ACETONIDE
(try-am-<u>sin</u>-oh-lone)

(Kenalog)

Purpose: treatment of severe inflammation caused by dermatologic disorders

• •

Diabetic Medications
Glucagonlike Peptide-1 Receptor Agonists

EXENATIDE
(ex-<u>en</u>-a-tide)

(Byetta, Bydureon)

Purpose: management of type 2 diabetes

SIDE EFFECTS

Epidermal thinning
Burning, dryness of skin
Allergic contact dermatitis

Hypopigmentation
Hyperglycemia

NURSING CONSIDERATIONS

- Topical glucocorticoid
- Apply only to affected areas; do not get in eyes
- Leave site uncovered or lightly covered
- Occlusive dressing is not recommended, systemic absorption may occur
- Do not use on weeping, denuded, or infected areas
- Avoid sunlight on affected areas
- Rx

• •

SIDE EFFECTS

Nausea, vomiting, diarrhea
Constipation
Injection site reactions

Hypoglycemia
Pancreatitis
Headache
Dizziness

Decreased appetite/ weight loss
Gastroesophageal reflux

NURSING CONSIDERATIONS

- subQ: give extended-release product once weekly without regard to food; give immediate-release product twice daily 30 minutes before a meal
- Extended-release version requires reconstitution just before administration
- Both products are refrigerated before use
- Do not use in patients with severe renal impairment or history of pancreatitis
- Routinely monitor blood glucose
- Rx

ACARBOSE
(ay-<u>car</u>-bose)

(Precose)

Purpose: management of type 2 diabetes

. . . .

GLIMEPIRIDE
(glye-<u>meh</u>-pi-ride)

(Amaryl)

Purpose: management of type 2 diabetes

SIDE EFFECTS

Abdominal pain
Diarrhea
Flatulence

NURSING CONSIDERATIONS

- Used alone or in combination with a sulfonylurea or insulin
- PO: take with first bite of each meal, med blood level peaks in 1 hour
- Recognize signs of hypoglycemia: weakness, hunger, dizziness, tremors, anxiety, tachycardia, hunger, sweating
- Measure short-term effectiveness with blood sugar 1 hour after meals
- Measure long-term effectiveness with glycosylated Hgb every 3 months for the first year
- Wear medical information tag
- Rx

• •

SIDE EFFECTS

Headache	Photosensitivity	Increased liver
Weakness, dizziness	Hepatotoxicity	enzymes
Drowsiness	Cholestatic jaundice	

NURSING CONSIDERATIONS

- Do not drink alcohol since it may produce a disulfiram reaction: nausea, headache, cramps, flushing, hypoglycemia
- Assess for symptoms of cholestatic jaundice: dark urine, pruritus, yellow sclera (rare)
- Take at breakfast or first main meal; onset 1–1.5 hours, peak 1–3 hours, duration 10–24 hours
- Have a quick source of sugar or a glucagon emergency kit available
- Do not crush, chew, or break extended-release tablet
- Cross allergy possible if allergic to sulfonamide
- Monitor blood sugars
- Wear medical information tag
- Rx

GLIPIZIDE

(glip-i-zide)

(Glucotrol)

Purpose: management of type 2 diabetes

• •

GLYBURIDE

(glye-byoo-ride)

(DiaBeta)

Purpose: management of type 2 diabetes

SIDE EFFECTS

Headache

Weakness, dizziness

Drowsiness

Photosensitivity

Increased liver enzymes

Cholestatic jaundice

NURSING CONSIDERATIONS

- Do not drink alcohol since it can produce a disulfiram reaction: nausea, headache, cramps, flushing, hypoglycemia
- Assess for symptoms of cholestatic jaundice: dark urine, pruritus, yellow sclera (rare)
- Take at breakfast; onset 1–1.5 hours, peak 1–3 hours, duration 10–24 hours
- Immediate-release: take 30 minutes before meals, since absorption is delayed by food
- Have a quick source of sugar or a glucagon emergency kit available
- May cause hemolytic anemia when used with sulfonylurea agents
- Monitor blood sugar
- Wear medical information tag
- Rx

• •

SIDE EFFECTS

Headache

Weakness, dizziness

Photosensitivity

GI disturbances

Allergic skin reactions

Thrombocytopenia

Cholestatic jaundice

Blurred vision

Increased liver enzymes

Hepatotoxicity

Joint pain

NURSING CONSIDERATIONS

- Assess for symptoms of cholestatic jaundice: dark urine, pruritus, yellow sclera (rare)
- Take at breakfast; onset 2–4 hours, peak 4 hours, duration 24 hours
- Have a quick source of sugar or a glucagon emergency kit available
- Monitor blood sugar
- Wear medical information tag
- Rx

METFORMIN HCL
(met-<u>for</u>-min)

(Glucophage)

Purpose: management of type 2 diabetes

• •

PIOGLITAZONE HCL
(pye-oh-<u>glit</u>-a-zone)

(Actos)

Purpose: management of type 2 diabetes

SIDE EFFECTS

Headache	Agitation	Lactic acidosis
Weakness, dizziness, drowsiness	Nausea, vomiting, diarrhea	Thrombocytopenia
		Rash

NURSING CONSIDERATIONS

- PO: twice a day with meals to decrease GI upset and provide best absorption; may also be taken as one dose
- Can crush tablets and mix with juice or soft foods for ease of swallowing
- Do not crush, chew, or break extended-release tablet
- Be aware of signs of lactic acidosis: hyperventilation, fatigue, malaise, chills, myalgia, sleepiness
- Have a quick source of sugar or a glucagon emergency kit available
- Monitor blood sugar
- Wear medical information tag
- Rx

· ·

SIDE EFFECTS

Headache	Muscle pain
Sinusitis	MI, heart failure
Respiratory infection	Hepatotoxicity

NURSING CONSIDERATIONS

- Take around the same time each day, once daily, with or without food
- Full therapeutic effects may require 2 or more weeks
- Use in conjunction with diet and exercise regimen
- May exacerbate CHF; monitor for edema and lung sounds
- August 2011, FDA issued alert: use of drug for more than 1 year is associated with increased risk of bladder cancer
- Rx

ROSIGLITAZONE MALEATE
(roe-si-glit-a-zone may-lee-ate)

(Avandi)

Purpose: management of type 2 diabetes

• •

SITAGLIPTIN
(sye-ta-glip-tin)

(Januvia)

Purpose: management of type 2 diabetes as monotherapy or in combination with other antidiabetic agents

SIDE EFFECTS

Headache, fatigue
MI, CHF
Weight gain

Hepatotoxicity
Increased
   cholesterol levels

URI, sinusitis
Back pain
Pulmonary edema

NURSING CONSIDERATIONS

- PO: once a day or in 2 divided doses
- Take without regard to meals
- Have a quick source of sugar or a glucagon emergency kit available
- Wear medical information tag
- Avoid OTC, herbals, nitrates, and insulin unless approved by provider
- Rx

* *

SIDE EFFECTS

Pancreatitis
Headache
Nausea, vomiting

Acute renal failure
Peripheral edema
Anaphylaxis

NURSING CONSIDERATIONS

- Take with or without food
- Do not split, crush, or chew
- Contact provider immediately if symptoms of pancreatitis: persistent, severe abdominal pain with or without vomiting
- Rx

INSULIN ASPART
(<u>in</u>-suh-lin <u>ass</u>-part)

(NovoLog)

Purpose: management of diabetes

• •

INSULIN GLARGINE
(<u>in</u>-suh-lin <u>glar</u>-jeen)

(Lantus, Lantus Solostar)

Purpose: management of diabetes

SIDE EFFECTS

Hypoglycemia   Allergic reactions   Blurred vision
Lipodystrophy   Headache   Flushing
Hypokalemia   Edema

NURSING CONSIDERATIONS

- The only insulin analog approved for use in external pump systems for continuous subQ insulin infusion
- Onset 15 minutes, peak 1–3 hours, duration 3–5 hours
- May be administered IV in emergency situations under medical supervision with close blood-sugar monitoring
- Immediately follow injection with meal within 5–10 minutes
- Rx

• •

SIDE EFFECTS

Hypoglycemia   Headache   Flushing
Lipodystrophy   Edema   Hypokalemia
Allergic reactions Blurred vision

NURSING CONSIDERATIONS

- No pronounced peak, duration 24 hours
- Must inject at same time each day
- Not the drug of choice for diabetic ketoacidosis (use a short-acting insulin)
- Higher incidence of injection site pain compared with NPH insulin
- Monitor blood sugar
- Do not administer IV or via insulin pump
- Do not mix with any other insulin
- Rx

INSULIN-ISOPHANE SUSPENSION (NPH)
(<u>in</u>-suh-lin <u>eye</u>-soe-fane)

(Humulin N, Novolin N)

Purpose: management of diabetes

. . . .

INSULIN LISPRO
(<u>in</u>-suh-lin <u>liss</u>-pro)

(Humalog)

Purpose: management of diabetes

SIDE EFFECTS

Hypoglycemia   Headache   Flushing
Lipodystrophy   Edema   Hypokalemia
Allergic reactions   Blurred vision

NURSING CONSIDERATIONS

- Comes in 100 units per milliliter vial, as well as in combination with regular insulin in a 50/50 proportion and 75/25 proportion
- subQ: onset 1–1.5 hours, peak 4–12 hours, duration 18–24 hours
- Read administration instructions carefully
- Do not give IV
- Monitor blood sugar
- OTC, Rx

• •

SIDE EFFECTS

Hypoglycemia   Edema
Lipodystrophy   Blurred vision
Allergic reactions   Hypokalemia
Headache

NURSING CONSIDERATIONS

- Take within 15 minutes of eating and immediately after mixing, with combined therapy
- May be used in children in combination with sulfonylureas
- Onset rapid, peak 30–90 minutes, duration 6–8 hours
- May be used in an external insulin pump
- Monitor blood sugar
- May be administered IV in emergency situations under medical supervision with close blood-sugar monitoring
- If administered using insulin pen, read instructions carefully
- Do not mix with other insulins
- Available in combination with other insulin
- Rx

INSULIN, REGULAR

(<u>in</u>-suh-lin)

(Humulin R)

Purpose: management of diabetes

· ·

GLUCAGON

(<u>gloo</u>-ka-gon)

(GlucaGen)

Purpose: acute management of hypoglycemia, facilitation of diagnostic tests through temporary inhibition of GI tract movement

SIDE EFFECTS

Hypoglycemia	Hypokalemia	Blurred vision
Lipodystrophy	Headache	Flushing
Allergic reaction	Edema	

NURSING CONSIDERATIONS

- Comes in 100 units/milliliter vial
- Only insulin that can be given IV in non-emergency situations
- subQ: onset 30–60 minutes, peak 2–3 hours, duration 3–6 hours
- IV: onset 10–30 minutes, peak 10–30 minutes, duration 30–60 minutes
- Read insulin pen instructions carefully
- May be mixed with NPH *only* in same syringe; draw regular insulin first
- Do not use in insulin pumps
- Monitor blood sugar
- Do not rub site after subQ injection
- OTC, Rx

• •

SIDE EFFECTS

Nausea, vomiting
Dizziness
Hypotension

NURSING CONSIDERATIONS

- IV: onset immediate, peak 30 minutes, duration 60–90 minutes
- subQ: onset within 10 minutes, peak 13–20 minutes, duration 30 minutes
- Monitor blood sugar until patient is asymptomatic
- Use reconstituted mixture within 15 minutes of mix
- OTC, Rx

ALUMINUM HYDROXIDE GEL
(uh-<u>loo</u>-min-um hye-<u>drok</u>-side)

(Amphojel)

Purpose: antacid; control of hyperphosphatemia in renal failure; adjunct therapy in ulcer treatment, GERD, and reflux esophagitis

• •

CALCIUM CARBONATE
(<u>kal</u>-see-um <u>kar</u>-buh-nate)

(Tums)

Purpose: antacid, calcium supplementation

SIDE EFFECTS

Constipation that
  may lead to
  impaction

Phosphate depletion
Hypomagnesemia
Hypercalciuria

NURSING CONSIDERATIONS

- PO: shake suspension well, follow with small amount of milk or water to facilitate passage; duration 20–180 minutes
- Contact provider if signs of GI bleeding: tarry stools, coffee-grounds vomitus
- Monitor long-term, high-dose use if on restricted sodium intake, due to high sodium content
- If prolonged use, monitor for phosphate depletion: anorexia, malaise, and muscle weakness; can also lead to resorption of calcium and bone demineralization in uremia patients
- Do not take longer than 2 weeks
- Rx

• •

SIDE EFFECTS

Nausea
Anorexia
Constipation
Dry mouth

Possible allergic
  reaction
Hypercalciuria

NURSING CONSIDERATIONS

- May decrease effect of some antibiotics and other drugs due to impaired absorption, so separate administration times by 2 hours
- Do not use if ventricular fibrillation or hypercalcemia
- Use caution if taking cardiac glycoside or has sarcoidosis or renal or cardiac disease
- Signs of hypercalcemia: nausea, vomiting, headache, confusion, anorexia
- OTC

Gastrointestinal Medications
Anticholinergics

HYOSCYAMINE
(hye-oh-<u>sye</u>-a-meen)

(Anaspaz, Gastrosed)

Purpose: treatment of peptic ulcer disease, other GI disorders, spastic disorders, IBS, and urinary incontinence

• •

Gastrointestinal Medications
Antidiarrheals

LOPERAMIDE HCL
(loe-<u>pair</u>-a-mide)

(Imodium)

Purpose: treatment of diarrhea and traveler's diarrhea

SIDE EFFECTS

Confusion, stimulation in elderly

Dry mouth, constipation

Urinary retention, hesitancy

Palpitations

Blurred vision, photophobia

Tachycardia

Rash

Headache

Drowsiness

NURSING CONSIDERATIONS

- PO: onset 20–30 minutes, duration 4–6 hours
- IM, IV, subQ: onset 2–3 minutes, duration 4–6 hours
- Avoid activities requiring alertness until stabilized on med
- Avoid alcohol, CNS depressants
- Take 30–60 minutes before meals
- Avoid antacids within 1 hour
- Rx

• •

SIDE EFFECTS

Nausea, vomiting

Abdominal pain/ distention

Dizziness

Drowsiness

Dry mouth

Rash

Hyperglycemia

NURSING CONSIDERATIONS

- Take with a full glass of water
- Encourage 6–8 glasses of fluid per day
- Use caution with potentially hazardous activities
- If abdominal distention in acute ulcerative colitis, stop med
- Avoid use with alcohol, CNS depressants
- Follow clear liquid or bland diet until diarrhea subsides
- Do not use OTC if fever over 101°F (38°C) or if bloody diarrhea
- Use for 48 hours only
- OTC, Rx

MECLIZINE
(<u>mek</u>-li-zeen)

(Antivert, Bonine)

Purpose: management of vertigo and motion sickness

• •

METOCLOPRAMIDE HCL
(met-oh-<u>kloe</u>-pra-mide)

(Reglan)

Purpose: prevention of nausea and vomiting induced by chemotherapy, radiation-delayed gastric emptying, and GERD

SIDE EFFECTS

Drowsiness

Dizziness

Hypotension

Urinary retention

Dry mouth

Blurred vision

NURSING CONSIDERATIONS

- Duration 8–14 hours
- Take 1 hour before traveling
- Avoid activities requiring alertness
- Avoid alcohol, CNS depressants
- May give without regard to food
- OTC, Rx

• •

SIDE EFFECTS

Drowsiness

Restlessness,
dystonia

Headache

Dry mouth

Suicidal ideation

Hypotension

Neutropenia

NURSING CONSIDERATIONS

- Prevention of nausea, vomiting induced by chemotherapy, radiation, delayed gastric emptying, GERD
- Used with tube feeding to decrease residual and risk of aspiration
- PO: take 30–60 minutes before meals or procedures
- IV: inject slowly over 1–2 minutes; infuse over 15 minutes
- Use caution with potentially hazardous activities
- Avoid alcohol, CNS depressants
- May cause tardive dyskinesia or neuroleptic malignant syndrome when used longer than 3 months
- May cause depression
- Rx

ONDANSETRON

(on-<u>don</u>-si-tron)

(Zofran)

Purpose: prevention of nausea and vomiting

• •

PROCHLORPERAZINE

(proe-klor-<u>pair</u>-a-zeen)

(Compro)

Purpose: treatment of nausea/vomiting and psychotic disorders

SIDE EFFECTS

Headache   Dry mouth
Dizziness, drowsiness   Bronchospasm
GI upset   Rash

NURSING CONSIDERATIONS

- Headache requiring analgesic is common
- Assess for extrapyramidal symptoms
- Rx

• •

SIDE EFFECTS

Orthostatic hypotension	Drowsiness, dizziness	Extrapyramidal symptoms
Blurred vision	Photosensitivity	Cholestatic jaundice
Dry mouth	Neuroleptic malignant syndrome	Leukopenia
Constipation		

NURSING CONSIDERATIONS

- Do not crush or break sustained-release capsules
- IM: inject slowly, deeply into gluteal muscle; keep patient lying down for 30 minutes
- Use caution with potentially hazardous activities
- Avoid changing positions (lying/sitting/standing) rapidly
- Check CBC and liver functions with prolonged use
- Risk of increase mortality in elderly patients with dementia; related psychosis
- Rx

PROMETHAZINE
(pro-<u>meth</u>-a-zeen)

(Phenergan)

Purpose: management of motion sickness, rhinitis, allergy symptoms, sedation, and nausea; pre- and postoperative sedation

• •

Gastrointestinal Medications
Antiflatulents

SIMETHICONE
(si-<u>meth</u>-i-kone)

(Gas-X, Mylanta)

Purpose: reduction of pressure and bloating caused by gas in digestive tract

SIDE EFFECTS

Drowsiness
Dizziness
Constipation
Urinary retention
Dry mouth

Hyperglycemia
Photosensitivity
Neuroleptic
  malignant
  syndrome

Hypo/hypertension
Blurred vision
Thrombocytopenia

NURSING CONSIDERATIONS

- PO: onset 20 minutes, duration 4–12 hours
- Take 30–60 minutes before traveling
- Avoid activities requiring alertness
- Avoid alcohol, CNS depressants
- May cause severe chemical irritation and damage to tissue when used IV
- May lower seizure threshold
- May cause false results in pregnancy testing
- Rx

• •

SIDE EFFECTS

Belching
Rectal flatus

NURSING CONSIDERATIONS

- Take after meals, at bedtime
- Shake suspension well before pouring
- Tablets must be chewed
- OTC, Rx

ESOMEPRAZOLE
(ess-oh-<u>meh</u>-pruh-zole)

(Nexium)

Purpose: treatment of GERD and severe erosive esophagitis

• •

OMEPRAZOLE
(oh-<u>meh</u>-pruh-zole)

(Prilosec)

*Purpose: treatment of GERD, severe erosive esophagitis, and active
  duodenal ulcers*

SIDE EFFECTS

Headache, dizziness	Dry mouth	Heart failure
Diarrhea	Hepatic failure	Hypoglycemia
Nausea	Rash	
Flatulence	Cough	

NURSING CONSIDERATIONS

- Take at least 60 minutes before meals
- Swallow capsules whole; do not chew
- May be taken in conjunction with antacids
- Rx

• •

SIDE EFFECTS

Headache, dizziness	Hepatic failure	URI, cough
Nausea, vomiting, diarrhea	Rash, urticaria	Electrolyte imbalances
Flatulence	Back pain	Hypoglycemia

NURSING CONSIDERATIONS

- Take 30 minutes before eating
- May be taken at the same time as antacids
- Avoid activities requiring alertness
- OTC, Rx

CIMETIDINE
(sye-<u>met</u>-uh-deen)

(Tagamet)

Purpose: treatment of ulcers and GERD, prevention of upper GI bleeding

• •

FAMOTIDINE
(fuh-<u>moe</u>-ti-deen)

(Pepcid)

Purpose: treatment of ulcers, GERD, and heartburn

SIDE EFFECTS

Diarrhea
Confusion (esp. in elderly with large doses)
Headache, dizziness

Dysrhythmias
Paralytic ileus
Agranulocytosis
Pneumonia
Rash

Impotence
Increased liver and renal enzymes

NURSING CONSIDERATIONS

- Reduces gastric acid secretions by 50–80%
- May be taken without regard to meals
- Avoid antacids 1 hour before or after dose
- Do not use OTC medications
- OTC, Rx

• •

SIDE EFFECTS

Headache
Hepatitis
Dizziness

Constipation
Dysrhythmias
Taste changes

Arthralgia
Nausea, vomiting

NURSING CONSIDERATIONS

- PO: onset 60 minutes, peak 1–3 hours, duration 6–12 hours
- IV: onset 60 minutes, peak 1–4 hours, duration 12 hours
- OTC, Rx

LANSOPRAZOLE
(lan-<u>soe</u>-pruh-zole)

(Prevacid)

Purpose: treatment of GERD, ulcers, and erosive esophagitis

• •

MISOPROSTOL
(mye-soe-<u>pross</u>-tole)

(Cytotec)

Purpose: prevention of gastric ulcers during NSAID therapy

SIDE EFFECTS

Dizziness
Constipation
Abdominal pain
Headache
Impotence

Kidney stones
Hematuria
Hypoglycemia
Altered hepatic lab
  values

NURSING CONSIDERATIONS

- PO: take 30 minutes before meals; capsules may be opened and sprinkled on food and swallowed immediately
- Can use with antacids
- Report severe diarrhea
- Rx

• •

SIDE EFFECTS

Abdominal pain
Diarrhea
Miscarriage

Nausea
Headache
Menstrual disorders

NURSING CONSIDERATIONS

- Take with meals and at bedtime
- Avoid taking magnesium antacids within 2 hours
- Notify provider if black, tarry stools, severe abdominal pain, or diarrhea
- Rx

PANTOPRAZOLE
(pan-<u>toe</u>-pruh-zole)

(Protonix)

Purpose: treatment of GERD and ulcers

. . . .

RABEPRAZOLE
(ruh-<u>bep</u>-ruh-zole)

(AcipHex)

Purpose: treatment of GERD and ulcers

SIDE EFFECTS

Headache
Insomnia
Fatigue
Abdominal pain
Diarrhea

Pancreatitis
Rash
Hyperglycemia
Weight changes
Hyponatremia

Hypomagnesemia
Muscle pain
Hyperglycemia

NURSING CONSIDERATIONS

- Take without regard to food
- Notify provider if black tarry stools, severe abdominal pain, or diarrhea
- Avoid alcohol, salicylates, NSAIDs
- Vitamin B12 deficiency may occur with long-term therapy
- Rx

• •

SIDE EFFECTS

Headache
Dizziness
Nausea, vomiting,
    diarrhea
Constipation,
    flatulence

Rash
Back pain
URI, proteinuria
Hypoglycemia
Chest pain,
    tachycardia

Diarrhea
Thrombocytopenia
URI, cough

NURSING CONSIDERATIONS

- Take without regard to food
- Swallow tablets whole; do not crush, chew, or split tablets
- Avoid alcohol, NSAIDs, and ASA; may increase gastric upset
- Vitamin B12 deficiency may occur with long-term therapy
- Report severe diarrhea or black stools immediately
- Rx

RANITIDINE
(ra-<u>nit</u>-i-deen)

(Zantac)

Purpose: inhibition of acid gastric secretions

• •

SUCRALFATE
(soo-<u>kral</u>-fate)

(Carafate)

Purpose: treatment of duodenal ulcers

SIDE EFFECTS

Dizziness (esp. in elderly)
Drowsiness
Headache

Tachycardia, PVCs
Blurred vision
Impotence
Hepatotoxicity

Constipation, abdominal pain
Pneumonia

NURSING CONSIDERATIONS

- Take without regard to meals
- Do not take antacids within 1 hour before or after medication
- Do not smoke; it interferes with healing and drug's effectiveness
- Avoid alcohol, ASA, and caffeine, which increase stomach acid
- False positive tests for urine protein may occur
- OTC, Rx

• •

SIDE EFFECTS

Constipation
Drowsiness, dizziness
Dry mouth

Rash, urticaria
Hyperglycemia

NURSING CONSIDERATIONS

- PO: 1 hour before meals or 2 hours after meals and at bedtime with full glass of water
- Do not chew or crush tablets
- Do not use antacids within 30 minutes of med
- Encourage 8–10 glasses of fluid per day
- Avoid smoking
- Not to be used for longer than 8 weeks
- Rx

SULFASALAZINE
(sul-fuh-<u>sal</u>-a-zeen)

(Azulfidine)

Purpose: treatment of ulcerative colitis and rheumatoid arthritis

• •

PHENTERMINE
(<u>fen</u>-tur-meen)

(Adipex-P, Suprenza, Zantryl)

Purpose: short-term appetite suppression

SIDE EFFECTS

Headache, confusion

Nausea, vomiting, diarrhea

Rashes
Fever
Hepatotoxicity
Renal failure

Photosensitivity
Leukopenia
Rash, urticaria

NURSING CONSIDERATIONS

- PO: take with food to decrease GI upset
- Encourage fluids to decrease crystallization in kidneys
- May stain contact lenses, urine, and skin yellow
- Rx

• •

SIDE EFFECTS

CNS stimulation
Hyper/hypotension
Impotence
Palpitations

Drowsiness, nervousness

Dry mouth, altered taste

Bone marrow suppression

Rash, urticaria
Shortness of breath

NURSING CONSIDERATIONS

- PO, hydrochloride form: duration 4 hours
- PO, resin complex form: duration 12–14 hours
- Take 30 minutes before meals or as a single dose before breakfast or 10–14 hours before bedtime
- Avoid activities requiring alertness until response is known
- Avoid alcohol, CNS depressants
- Contact provider if chest pain, decreased exercise tolerance, fainting, or lower extremity swelling
- Monitor weight 3 times per week
- Rx C-IV

LACTULOSE
(lak-tyoo-lose)

(Cephulac, Chronulac)

Purpose: relief of chronic constipation, prevention and treatment of portal-systemic encephalopathy

• •

PANCRELIPASE
(pan-kre-li-pase)

(Pancrease, Viokase)

Purpose: treatment of exocrine pancreatic secretion insufficiency and pancreatic enzyme deficiency, digestive aid for cystic fibrosis

SIDE EFFECTS

Nausea, vomiting
Abdominal cramps,
  distention
Hypernatremia

NURSING CONSIDERATIONS

- PO: take with water or fruit juice to counteract sweet taste
- Use with caution in diabetics
- Rx

. . . .

SIDE EFFECTS

Abdominal pain (high doses only)	Stomach cramps	Hypo/hyperglycemia
Nausea, diarrhea	Abnormal feces	Hyperuricemia
	Fatigue	

NURSING CONSIDERATIONS

- Take with 8 oz water and food, swallow right away, sit up when taking
- Do not use if sensitive or allergy to pork
- Stools will be foul-smelling and frothy
- Rx

TAMSULOSIN HCL
(tam-<u>soo</u>-luh-sin)

(Flomax)

Purpose: treatment benign prostatic hyperplasia

. . . .

OXYBUTYNIN CHLORIDE
(ox-ee-<u>byoo</u>-ti-nin <u>klor</u>-ide)

(Ditropan)

Purpose: antispasmodic for neurogenic bladder and overactive bladder in females

SIDE EFFECTS

Insomnia

Nausea, vomiting, diarrhea

Blurred vision

Abnormal ejaculation, priapism

Dizziness

Headache

Increased cough

Chest pain, orthostatic hypertension

Floppy iris syndrome

NURSING CONSIDERATIONS

- Take the same time daily, once a day, 30 minutes after a meal
- Avoid changing positions (lying, sitting, standing) rapidly
- Use caution in potentially hazardous activities
- This medication should be stopped prior to cataract surgery; may cause floppy iris syndrome
- Do not crush, break, or chew capsules
- Rx

• •

SIDE EFFECTS

Anxiety, restlessness

Dizziness

Seizures

Palpitations, tachycardia

Drowsiness, blurred vision

Nausea, vomiting

Anorexia

Dry mouth

Constipation

Hypertension

Impotence

Angioedema

NURSING CONSIDERATIONS

- Take without regard to meals
- Avoid alcohol, CNS depressants
- Avoid activities requiring alertness until med response is known
- Decreased ability to perspire; avoid strenuous activity in warm weather
- Rx, OTC

TOLTERODINE TARTRATE
(tol-<u>tair</u>-uh-deen)
(Detrol, Detrol LA)

Purpose: treatment of overactive bladder and urinary incontinence

• •

Genitourinary Medications
Erectile Dysfunction Agents

SILDENAFIL CITRATE
(sil-<u>den</u>-a-fill <u>sih</u>-trate)
(Viagra)

Purpose: treatment of erectile dysfunction

SIDE EFFECTS

Dry mouth
Dizziness, headache
Constipation
Nausea, vomiting
Dyspepsia
Blurred vision

UTI
Hepatic injury
Chest pain, hypertension
Anxiety
Rash, pruritus
URI, cough

NURSING CONSIDERATIONS

- Patients should avoid alcohol during treatment
- Take without regard to meals
- Rx

• •

SIDE EFFECTS

Headache, flushing
Dizziness
Nasal congestion

UTI
Abnormal vision
Rash

Tinnitus, hearing loss
Visual disturbances

NURSING CONSIDERATIONS

- Take approximately 1 hour before sexual activity
- Do not use more than once a day
- Tablets may be split
- High-fat meal will reduce absorption; better absorption on empty stomach
- Never use with nitrates; could have fatal fall in blood pressure
- Notify provider if erection lasts longer than 4 hours
- Stop medication if hearing or visual disturbances occur
- Does not protect against sexually transmitted diseases
- Rx

TADALAFIL
(tuh-<u>dal</u>-uh-fill)

(Cialis)

Purpose: treatment of erectile dysfunction and benign prostatic hyperplasia

• •

VARDENAFIL
(var-<u>den</u>-uh-fill)

(Levitra)

Purpose: treatment of erectile dysfunction

SIDE EFFECTS

Headache, flushing	Tinnitus, hearing loss	Hypotension
Dyspepsia	Nasal congestion	UTI
Back pain	Dizziness	Blurred vision

NURSING CONSIDERATIONS

- Take 1 hour before sexual activity
- Take at same time each day for BPH
- Patients with severe hepatic impairment should not take
- Alert provider if erection lasts more than 4 hours
- Stop medication if hearing or visual disturbances occur
- Alcohol intake may increase orthostatic symptoms
- Never use with nitrates; could have fatal fall in BP
- Does not protect against sexually transmitted diseases
- Rx

• •

SIDE EFFECTS

Headache, dizziness	Tinnitus, hearing loss	Photophobia
Nasal congestion		Arthralgia
Flushing	Hypertension, chest pain	Sinusitis
Dyspepsia, GERD		

NURSING CONSIDERATIONS

- Take 1 hour before sexual activity
- Contact provider if erection lasts over 4 hours
- Stop medication if hearing or visual disturbances occur
- Never use with nitrates; could have fatal fall in BP
- Does not protect against sexually transmitted diseases
- Rx

FINASTERIDE
(fuh-<u>nas</u>-tuh-ride)

(Proscar, Propecia)

Purpose: treatment of benign prostatic hyperplasia (Proscar) and male pattern baldness (Propecia)

• •

Genitourinary Medications
Urinary Analgesics

PHENAZOPYRIDINE HCL
(fen-<u>az</u>-uh-<u>peer</u>-i-deen)

(Pyridium)

Purpose: treatment of urinary tract irritation (often in combination with urinary anti-infective)

SIDE EFFECTS

Decreased libido

Decreased volume of
  ejaculate

Testicular pain

Impotence

Breast tenderness and
  enlargement

Decreased PSA levels

NURSING CONSIDERATIONS

- May be taken without regard to food
- Pregnant women should avoid contact with crushed drug or patient's semen; may adversely affect developing male fetus
- Full therapeutic effect: Propecia may require 3 months, Proscar may require 6–12 months
- Not for use in women and children
- Rx

• •

SIDE EFFECTS

GI upset

Kidney and liver toxicity

Rash

Headache, vertigo

NURSING CONSIDERATIONS

- Do not crush tablets; can take with food or milk to decrease GI upset
- Inform patient that urine will be bright orange/red
- Monitor for signs of hepatoxicity: dark urine, clay-colored stools, jaundice, itching, abdominal pain, fever, diarrhea
- May interfere with urine glucose tests
- OTC, Rx

NITROFURANTOIN
(<u>nye</u>-troe-fyoo-<u>ran</u>-tuh-win)

(Furadantin, Macrobid, Macrodantin)

Purpose: treatment of urinary tract infection

• •

Hormones/Synthetic Substitutes/Modifiers
Bone Resorption Inhibitors

ALENDRONATE
(al-en-<u>drone</u>-ate)

(Fosamax)

Purpose: treatment and prevention of osteoporosis and Paget disease

SIDE EFFECTS

Dizziness, headache

Nausea, vomiting, diarrhea

Abdominal pain

Tooth staining

Chills, confusion

Rash, pruritus

Chest pain

Hepatitis

Pancreatitis

Anemia

Cough, dyspnea

NURSING CONSIDERATIONS

- Take with food or milk
- Two daily doses if urine output is high or patient has diabetes
- Drug may turn urine rust-yellow to brown
- May cause false positive glucose in urine
- Do not break, crush, chew, or open tablets or capsules
- Rx

• •

SIDE EFFECTS

Esophageal ulceration

GI distress

Musculoskeletal pain, bone fractures

Hypophosphatemia

Hypocalcemia

Angioedema

NURSING CONSIDERATIONS

- Onset: 1 month, peak 3–6 months, duration 3 weeks to 7 months
- Take in a.m. before food or other meds with full glass of water; remain upright for 30 minutes
- If dose missed, skip dose; do not double dose or take later in the day
- Take with calcium and vitamin D if instructed by provider
- Rx

CALCITONIN
(kal-suh-<u>toe</u>-nin)

(Miacalcin)

Purpose: treatment of hypercalcemia, Paget disease, and osteoporosis

• •

Hormones/Synthetic Substitutes/Modifiers
Bone Resorption Inhibitors

RISEDRONATE
(riss-<u>ed</u>-ruh-nate)

(Actonel)

Purpose: prevention and treatment of osteoporosis and Paget disease

SIDE EFFECTS

Headache

Weakness, dizziness

Chest pressure, hypertension

Nasal congestion

Nausea, vomiting, diarrhea

Abdominal pain

Salty taste

Diuresis, nocturia

Flushing

Myalgia, tingling of hands

Dyspnea, bronchospasms

NURSING CONSIDERATIONS

- subQ: give at bedtime to minimize nausea and vomiting, rotate injection sites
- IM: give only with epinephrine emergency medications
- IM/subQ: onset 15 minutes, peak 4 hours
- Rx

• •

SIDE EFFECTS

Weakness, headache

Diarrhea, abdominal pain

Bone, back, joint pain

UTI

Fractures

Chest pain, hypertension

Hypocalcemia

Hypophosphatemia

NURSING CONSIDERATIONS

- Onset: within days, peak 30 days, duration up to 16 months
- Take in a.m. before food or other meds with full glass of water; remain upright for 30 minutes
- Take with calcium and vitamin D if instructed by provider
- Rx

Hormones/Synthetic Substitutes/Modifiers
Thyroid Hormones

LEVOTHYROXINE (T4)
(lee-voe-thye-<u>rox</u>-een)

(Synthroid, Levothroid)

Purpose: management of hypothyroidism and myxedema coma

• •

Mental Health Medications
Antianxiety Agents

ALPRAZOLAM
(al-<u>praz</u>-uh-lam)

(Xanax)

Purpose: management of anxiety and panic disorders

SIDE EFFECTS

Weight loss

Arrhythmias, tachycardia

Insomnia, irritability

Nervousness

Heat intolerance

Menstrual irregularities

Thyroid storm

Hypertension

NURSING CONSIDERATIONS

- PO: onset 24 hours
- PO: take at same time daily to maintain blood level; take on empty stomach
- Do not switch brands unless directed
- Avoid OTC meds with iodine and iodized salt, soybeans, tofu, turnips, walnuts, some seafood, some bread
- Medication controls symptoms and treatment is lifelong
- Separate antacids, iron, and calcium products by 4 hours
- Rx

• •

SIDE EFFECTS

Dizziness, drowsiness

Orthostatic hypotension

Blurred vision

Memory impairment

Increased appetite

Suicidal ideation

Constipation, dry mouth

Decreased libido

NURSING CONSIDERATIONS

- Onset 30 minutes, peak 1–2 hours, duration 4–6 hours
- Full therapeutic response takes 2–3 days
- May be taken with food
- May be habit-forming; do not take for longer than 4 months unless directed
- Memory impairment is a sign of long-term use
- Do not stop med abruptly; may cause seizures
- Drowsiness may worsen at beginning of treatment
- Rx C-IV

BUSPIRONE

(byoo-<u>spye</u>-rone)

(BuSpar)

Purpose: management of anxiety disorders

• •

CHLORDIAZEPOXIDE

(<u>klor</u>-dye-az-uh-<u>pock</u>-side)

(Librium)

Purpose: management of anxiety and alcohol withdrawal

SIDE EFFECTS

Dizziness, headache
Insomnia, nervousness
Depression
Lightheadedness, numbness

Nausea, diarrhea, constipation
Tachycardia, palpitations
Change in libido
Hyper/hypotension

Blurred vision
Sore throat
SOB, chest congestion

NURSING CONSIDERATIONS

- Onset 7–10 days, optimum effect may take 3–4 weeks
- Use caution with activities requiring alertness until response to med is known
- Avoid alcohol, CNS depressants, and grapefruit juice
- Use caution when changing positions because fainting may occur, especially in elderly
- Drowsiness may worsen at beginning of treatment
- Rx

• •

SIDE EFFECTS

Dizziness
Drowsiness
Pain at IM site
Disorientation
Orthostatic hypotension

Tachycardia
Blurred vision
Decreased libido
Rash

NURSING CONSIDERATIONS

- PO: onset 30 minutes, peak 2 hours
- IM: onset 15–30 minutes, slow, erratic absorption
- IV: onset 1–5 minutes, duration 15–60 minutes
- Use caution with activities requiring alertness until response to med is known
- Abrupt stop may lead to withdrawal: insomnia, irritability, nervousness, tremors
- Avoid alcohol, CNS depressants
- Tablets may be crushed and taken with food or fluids for ease of swallowing
- Rx C-IV

DIAZEPAM

(dye-<u>az</u>-uh-pam)

(Valium)

Purpose: management of anxiety, alcohol withdrawal, and seizure disorders; relaxation of skeletal muscle; preoperative sedation

• •

LORAZEPAM

(lor-<u>az</u>-uh-pam)

(Ativan)

Purpose: management of anxiety and irritability in psychiatric disorders, treatment of insomnia, adjunct therapy for endoscopic procedures, relief of preoperative anxiety

SIDE EFFECTS

Drowsiness, fatigue, ataxia

Paradoxic anxiety, esp. in elderly

Orthostatic hypotension

Blurred vision

Constipation, dry mouth

Neutropenia

Respiratory depression

NURSING CONSIDERATIONS

- PO: may be taken with food, onset 30 minutes, peak 2 hours
- IM: inject deep, slowly into large muscle mass; onset 15–30 minutes, duration 60–90 minutes, slow and erratic absorption
- IV: into large vein, push doses should not exceed 5 mg/minute, resuscitation equipment available; onset immediate, duration 15 minutes to 1 hour
- Smoking may decrease effectiveness
- Avoid use with alcohol, CNS depressants
- May be habit-forming if used longer than 4 months
- Do not discontinue abruptly after long-term use
- Rx C-IV

• •

SIDE EFFECTS

Dizziness, drowsiness

Orthostatic hypotension

Blurred vision

Weakness, headache

Disorientation

Constipation, dry mouth

Rash, dermatitis

Acidosis

NURSING CONSIDERATIONS

- PO: onset 1 hour, peak 2 hours
- IM: onset 15–30 minutes, peak 60–90 minutes
- IV: onset 5–15 minutes, peak 60–90 minutes
- May be taken with food
- May be habit-forming; do not take for longer than 4 months unless directed
- Avoid alcohol, CNS depressants
- Do not stop drug abruptly after long-term use
- Drowsiness may worsen at beginning of treatment
- Rx C-IV

CITALOPRAM
(sye-<u>tal</u>-uh-pram)

(Celexa)

Purpose: treatment of major depression

• •

ESCITALOPRAM OXALATE
(es-suh-<u>tal</u>-uh-pram <u>ox</u>-a-late)

(Lexapro)

Purpose: treatment of major depression and anxiety

SIDE EFFECTS

Palpitations, tachycardia
Orthostatic hypotension
Decreased appetite

Nausea, vomiting, diarrhea
Nervousness
Drowsiness
Hyponatremia
Sweating

Cough, bronchitis
Headache
Visual changes
Dry mouth
UTI
Decreased libido

NURSING CONSIDERATIONS

- Take consistently at same time of day; therapeutic effects in up to 4 weeks
- Take at bedtime if oversedation occurs during day
- Can potentiate effects of digoxin, warfarin, and diazepam
- Avoid use with alcohol, CNS depressants
- Use caution in potentially hazardous activities
- Avoid changing positions (lying, sitting, standing) rapidly
- May increase risk of suicidal thoughts and behavior
- May cause serotonin syndrome
- Rx

● ●

SIDE EFFECTS

Nausea, diarrhea, constipation
Fatigue, drowsiness
Decreased libido, sexual dysfunction
Nasal congestion, cough

Dry mouth
Dizziness, headache
Hypokalemia
Hyponatremia
Visual disturbances
Pain, arthritis
Sweating, rash

Hot flashes, palpitations
Postural hypotension
Hepatitis
Impaired platelet aggregation

NURSING CONSIDERATIONS

- Take consistently at same time of day; therapeutic effect in up to 4 weeks
- May require gradual reduction before stopping
- Can potentiate effects of digoxin, warfarin, diazepam
- Use caution in potentially hazardous activities; avoid alcohol
- May increase risk of suicidal thoughts or behaviors
- Teach patient to avoid aspirin and NSAIDs due to increased bleeding risk
- May cause serotonin syndrome
- Rx

FLUOXETINE HCL
(floo-<u>ox</u>-uh-teen)

(Prozac)

Purpose: treatment of major depression, OCD, bulimia, premenstrual dysphoric disorder, and panic disorders

• •

PAROXETINE HCL
(pa-<u>rox</u>-uh-teen)

(Paxil)

Purpose: treatment of depressive disorders, OCD, panic disorders, anxiety, PTSD, premenstrual disorders, and social anxiety

SIDE EFFECTS

Palpitations, hot flashes

Nausea, diarrhea, constipation

Decreased appetite

Nervousness, insomnia

UTI, frequency

Drowsiness, headache

Rash, pruritus, excessive sweating

Fatigue

Tachycardia

Visual changes

Hemorrhage

Hyponatremia

Cough, dyspnea

NURSING CONSIDERATIONS

- Take consistently at same time of day; full therapeutic effects may require 4 weeks
- Can potentiate effects of digoxin, warfarin, diazepam, NSAIDs, and aspirin
- Avoid use with alcohol, CNS depressants
- Use caution in potentially hazardous activities
- May increase risk of suicidal thoughts or behavior
- May cause serotonin syndrome
- Rx

• •

SIDE EFFECTS

Palpitations, postural hypotension

Nervousness, insomnia

Nausea, vomiting, diarrhea, constipation

Hyponatremia

Decreased appetite

Impotence

UTI

Sweating

Nasal congestion, cough

NURSING CONSIDERATIONS

- Decreases digoxin levels
- Take consistently at same time of day; full therapeutic effects may require 4 weeks
- Take with food or milk to reduce GI symptoms
- May increase risk of suicidal thoughts or behavior
- May increase risk of bleeding
- Avoid use with alcohol, CNS depressants
- Use caution in potentially hazardous activities
- Do not discontinue abruptly
- May cause serotonin syndrome
- Rx

SERTRALINE HCL
(<u>sur</u>-truh-leen)

(Zoloft)

Purpose: treatment of major depression, OCD, PTSD, panic disorder, social anxiety disorder, and premenstrual dysphoric disorder

• •

AMITRIPTYLINE
(a-muh-<u>trip</u>-tuh-leen)

Purpose: treatment of major depression

SIDE EFFECTS

Headache, agitation
Dizziness, confusion
Tremor
Nausea, diarrhea
Sweating

Insomnia
Dry mouth
Male sexual
   dysfunction
Palpitations

Vision abnormalities
SIADH
Hepatitis
Hyponatremia

NURSING CONSIDERATIONS

- Take consistently at same time of day; full therapeutic effect may require 4 weeks
- Take with food or milk to reduce GI symptoms
- Can potentiate effects of digoxin, warfarin, diazepam, aspirin, and NSAIDs
- Avoid use with alcohol, CNS depressants, and disulfiram
- Use caution in potentially hazardous activities
- May increase risk of suicidal thoughts or behavior
- May cause serotonin syndrome
- Rx

. . . .

SIDE EFFECTS

Sedation/drowsiness
Blurred vision,
   dry mouth,
   diaphoresis
Nausea, vomiting,
   diarrhea
Photosensitivity

Constipation,
   urinary retention
Increased appetite
Sexual dysfunction
Confusion
Tachycardia,
   dysrhythmias

Orthostatic
   hypotension
Hepatitis
Thrombocytopenia
Asthma
   exacerbation

NURSING CONSIDERATIONS

- Suicide risk high after 10–14 days due to increased energy
- Use safety precautions with hazardous activity
- Avoid use with alcohol
- Avoid sudden positional changes
- Do not discontinue abruptly
- May cause serotonin syndrome
- Rx

DOXEPIN
(<u>dox</u>-uh-pin)

Purpose: treatment of major depression and anxiety

• •

IMIPRAMINE
(im-<u>ip</u>-ruh-meen)

(Tofranil)

Purpose: treatment of depression and enuresis in children

SIDE EFFECTS

Sedation/
  drowsiness
Blurred vision,
  dry mouth,
  diaphoresis
Nausea, vomiting,
  diarrhea

Agranulocytosis
Constipation,
  urinary retention
Sexual dysfunction
Headache,
  confusion
Photosensitivity

Orthostatic
  hypotension
Palpitations,
  dysrhythmias
Paralytic ileus
Hepatitis
Acute renal failure

NURSING CONSIDERATIONS

- Full therapeutic effect may require 2–3 weeks
- Suicide risk high after 10–14 days due to increased energy
- Use safety precautions with hazardous activity
- Avoid use with alcohol, CNS depressants
- Avoid sudden positional changes
- Do not discontinue abruptly
- May worsen depression
- Rx

• •

SIDE EFFECTS

Sedation/drowsiness
Dry mouth
Acute renal failure
Photosensitivity
Hyperglycemia
Diarrhea

Urinary retention
Agranulocytosis
Confusion
Weight gain
Hyper/
  hypothyroidism

Orthostatic
  hypotension
Dysrhythmias
Blurred vision
Hepatitis

NURSING CONSIDERATIONS

- Drug is dispensed in small amounts at beginning of treatment
  due to suicide potential
- Full therapeutic effect may take 2–3 weeks
- Use safety precautions with hazardous activity
- Avoid sudden positional changes
- Avoid alcohol, CNS depressants
- Do not stop abruptly: could cause nausea, malaise, headache
- Rx

NORTRIPTYLINE

(nor-<u>trip</u>-tuh-leen)

(Pamelor)

Purpose: treatment of major depression

• •

BUPROPION HCL

(byoo-<u>proe</u>-pee-on)

(Wellbutrin, Zyban)

Purpose: treatment of depression (Wellbutrin), smoking cessation (Zyban)

SIDE EFFECTS

Sedation/drowsiness
Blurred vision, dry mouth, diaphoresis
Photosensitivity
Nausea, vomiting, diarrhea

Agranulocytosis
Constipation, urinary retention
Increased appetite
Sexual dysfunction
Dysrhythmias
SIADH

Acute renal failure
Hepatitis
Orthostatic hypotension
Hyponatremia
Hypothyroidism

NURSING CONSIDERATIONS

- Full therapeutic effect may require 2–3 weeks
- Suicide risk high after 10–14 days due to increased energy
- Use safety precautions with hazardous activity
- Avoid use with alcohol, CNS depressants
- Avoid sudden positional changes
- Do not stop abruptly
- May cause serotonin syndrome
- Rx

• •

SIDE EFFECTS

Agitation
Nausea, vomiting
Headache
Dry mouth
Weight loss/gain

Impotence
Tremor
Nervousness
Rash
Dysrhythmias

Hyper/hypotension
Blurred vision
Auditory disturbances

NURSING CONSIDERATIONS

- If missed dose for depression, take as soon as possible and space remaining doses at not less than 4-hour intervals
- If missed dose for smoking cessation, omit dose
- Taper dose before stopping
- Avoid use with alcohol, CNS depressants
- Use caution in potentially hazardous activities
- Avoid sudden positional changes
- May increase risk for suicidal thoughts or behavior
- Rx

DULOXETINE HCL

(doo-<u>lox</u>-uh-teen)

(Cymbalta)

Purpose: treatment of major depression, neuropathic pain, anxiety, fibromyalgia, and chronic lower back pain

• •

MIRTAZAPINE

(mer-<u>taz</u>-uh-peen)

(Remeron)

Purpose: treatment of depression

SIDE EFFECTS

Nausea, vomiting, diarrhea, constipation

Decreased appetite, stomach pain

Dry mouth

Hepatic failure

Increased urination, difficulty urinating

Dizziness, headache

Muscle spasms

Sexual dysfunction

Photosensitivity

Orthostatic hypotension

Palpitations

Thrombophlebitis

Hypo/hyperglycemia

NURSING CONSIDERATIONS

- Full therapeutic effect may require 4 weeks
- Taper dose before stopping
- Avoid sudden positional changes
- Avoid use with alcohol
- Use caution in potentially hazardous activities
- May increase risk of suicidal thoughts or behaviors
- Teach patient to avoid aspirin, NSAIDs (increased bleeding risk)
- May cause serotonin syndrome
- Rx

• •

SIDE EFFECTS

Drowsiness, dizziness

Increased appetite, weight gain

Constipation

Flulike symptoms

Dry mouth

Orthostatic hypotension

Palpitations

Blurred vision

Hepatitis

Renal failure

Agranulocytosis

Photosensitivity

NURSING CONSIDERATIONS

- Take without regard to food
- Do not use within 14 days of MAOI
- Therapeutic effect may take 2–3 weeks
- Taper dose before stopping
- Check with provider before taking OTC cold remedy
- Avoid alcohol, CNS depressants for up to 1 week after therapy
- Use caution in potentially hazardous activities
- May increase risk for suicidal thoughts or behavior
- May cause serotonin syndrome
- Rx

TRAZODONE
(<u>traz</u>-uh-doan)

Purpose: treatment of depression

• •

VENLAFAXINE
(ven-luh-<u>fax</u>-een)

(Effexor, Effexor XR)

Purpose: treatment of depression, anxiety, and panic disorder

SIDE EFFECTS

Drowsiness

Hypotension, dizziness

Dry mouth

Nausea

Blurred vision, photosensitivity

Priapism

Constipation, urinary retention

Tachycardia

Acute renal failure

Hepatitis

Agranulocytosis

NURSING CONSIDERATIONS

- Take at same time each day, preferably at bedtime on empty stomach
- Therapeutic effect may take 2–3 weeks
- Avoid use with alcohol, CNS depressants
- Avoid changing positions (lying, sitting, standing) rapidly
- Use caution in potentially hazardous activities
- May increase risk of suicidal thoughts or behavior
- Taper dose before stopping
- May cause serotonin syndrome
- Rx

• •

SIDE EFFECTS

Abnormal dreams, insomnia

Anxiety, nervousness

Dizziness, weakness

Headache

Ear pain

Nausea

Bronchitis, dyspnea

Thrombocytopenia

Sexual dysfunction

Hypertension

Serotonin syndrome

Photosensitivity

Abnormal bleeding

Increased cholesterol

Tachycardia

Abnormal vision

Peripheral edema

Dysphagia

NURSING CONSIDERATIONS

- Take with food; extended-release tablets should be swallowed whole
- Taper dose before stopping if taken over 6 weeks
- Avoid use with alcohol, CNS depressants for up to 1 week after end of therapy
- Use caution in potentially hazardous activities
- May increase risk of suicidal thoughts or behavior
- Rx

HALOPERIDOL

(hal-oh-<u>pair</u>-i-doll)

(Haldol)

Purpose: treatment of Tourette syndrome and schizophrenia, emergency sedation of severely agitated or delirious patients

. . . .

OLANZAPINE

(oh-<u>lan</u>-zuh-peen)

(Zyprexa)

Purpose: treatment of schizophrenia and manic episodes in bipolar disorder

SIDE EFFECTS

Drowsiness
Dizziness
Dyspnea
Urinary retention
Tachycardia

Hypotension
Confusion
Rash
Impotence
Photosensitivity

Hepatitis
Nausea, vomiting,
  dry mouth
Extrapyramidal
  symptoms

NURSING CONSIDERATIONS

- PO concentrate: dilute with water, not coffee or tea
- PO: take with food or full glass of water/milk
- IM: inject slowly, deep into large muscle; have patient lie down for 30 minutes; do not give IV
- Avoid abrupt withdrawal; discontinue gradually
- Avoid use with alcohol, CNS depressants
- Use caution in potentially hazardous activities
- Avoid changing positions (lying/sitting/standing) rapidly
- Wear protective clothing, sunglasses due to photosensitivity
- May cause neuroleptic malignant or serotonin syndrome
- Rx

• •

SIDE EFFECTS

Hostility
Dizziness
Rhinitis
Cough, pharyngitis
Nervousness
Joint pain
Dry mouth
Headache

Urinary retention
Insomnia
Increased appetite
  and weight gain
Fatigue
Impotence
Hyperlipidemia

Extrapyramidal
  symptoms
Heart failure
Hypo/hyperglycemia
Neutropenia
Orthostatic
  hypotension

NURSING CONSIDERATIONS

- Avoid changing positions rapidly
- Dosage should be managed tightly when established
- Use caution when operating equipment
- Avoid OTC preparations unless approved by provider
- May cause neuroleptic syndrome
- Rx

RISPERIDONE

(riss-<u>pair</u>-i-doan)

(Risperdal)

Purpose: treatment of schizophrenia, bipolar disorder, and irritability associated with autism

• •

QUETIAPINE

(kweh-<u>tye</u>-a-peen)

(Seroquel)

Purpose: treatment of bipolar disorder, depression, and schizophrenia

SIDE EFFECTS

Drowsiness
Dizziness
Headache, insomnia
Constipation
Hyperglycemia
Orthostatic hypotension

Extrapyramidal symptoms
Neuroleptic malignant
  syndrome
Heart failure
Neutropenia
URI

NURSING CONSIDERATIONS

- Avoid use with alcohol, CNS depressants
- Use caution in potentially hazardous activities
- Avoid changing positions (lying/sitting/standing) rapidly
- Avoid strenuous exercise in hot weather
- Avoid OTC meds unless approved by provider
- Rx

. . . .

SIDE EFFECTS

Drowsiness
Dizziness
Hyperglycemia
Nausea, anorexia
Dry mouth

Orthostatic
  hypotension
Agranulocytosis
Extrapyramidal
  symptoms

Hyperglycemia
SIADH
Hyponatremia
Back pain

NURSING CONSIDERATIONS

- Avoid use with alcohol, CNS depressants
- Use caution in potentially hazardous activities
- Avoid changing positions (lying/sitting/standing) rapidly
- Avoid strenuous exercise in hot weather
- Avoid OTC meds unless approved by provider
- May increase the risk of suicidal thoughts or behavior
- May cause neuroleptic malignant syndrome
- Rx

ZIPRASIDONE HCL

(zye-<u>praz</u>-i-doan)

(Geodon)

Purpose: treatment of schizophrenia, acute agitation, acute psychosis, bipolar disorder, and psychotic depression

• •

ARIPIPRAZOLE

(air-i-<u>pip</u>-ruh-zole)

(Abilify)

Purpose: treatment of schizophrenia, bipolar disorder, and major depressive disorder

SIDE EFFECTS

Drowsiness
Dizziness
Diarrhea
Abnormal vision
Vomiting, anorexia
Headache

Hyperglycemia
Orthostatic
    hypotension
Heart failure
Extrapyramidal
    symptoms

Impotence
Decreased bone
    density
Rhinitis, dyspnea

NURSING CONSIDERATIONS

- Avoid use with alcohol, CNS depressants
- Use caution in potentially hazardous activities
- Avoid changing positions (lying/sitting/standing) rapidly
- Avoid strenuous exercise in hot weather
- Check before taking OTC meds
- May cause neuroleptic malignant syndrome
- Rx

• •

SIDE EFFECTS

Headache
Insomnia
Anxiety
Cough
Weight gain
Hyperglycemia

Musculoskeletal
    pain
Nausea
Vomiting
Orthostatic
    hypotension

Neuroleptic
    malignant
    syndrome
Chest pain
Blurred vision
Rash

NURSING CONSIDERATIONS

- IM: inject deep, slowly into muscle mass; peak 1–3 hours
- PO: can take without regard to food; peak 3–5 hours
- Monitor for suicidal ideation
- Do not stop abruptly
- Rx

AMPHETAMINE/ DEXTROAMPHETAMINE

(am-<u>fet</u>-uh-meen/<u>decks</u>-troe-am-<u>fet</u>-uh-meen)

(Adderall, Adderall XR)

Purpose: treatment of ADHD and narcolepsy

• •

METHYLPHENIDATE HCL

(meth-ill-<u>fen</u>-uh-date)

(Concerta, Ritalin)

Purpose: treatment of ADD/ADHD in children over 6 years old, treatment of narcolepsy

SIDE EFFECTS

Headache, dizziness
Weight loss
Abdominal pain
Mood changes

Tachycardia
Insomnia
Dry mouth

NURSING CONSIDERATIONS

- Take in the morning
- High potential for abuse
- Rx C-II

• •

SIDE EFFECTS

Headache
Fever, arthralgia
Visual disturbance
Abdominal pain
Nausea, anorexia

Insomnia
Restlessness
Urticaria, rash
Leukopenia
Growth retardation

NURSING CONSIDERATIONS

- Concerta is time-released and should be swallowed whole, not chewed
- Dosage is adjusted in 18-mg increments to a maximum of 54 mg/day
- Avoid alcohol, caffeine, and OTC preparations
- Do not stop abruptly; taper over several weeks
- Monitor for adverse psychiatric symptoms
- Rx C-II

CARBAMAZEPINE
(kar-buh-<u>maz</u>-uh-peen)

(Tegretol, Tegretol XR)

Purpose: management of seizures, trigeminal neuralgia, and bipolar disorder

• •

LITHIUM
(<u>lith</u>-ee-um)

(Lithobid)

Purpose: management of manic phase in bipolar disorder, prevention of bipolar manic-depressive psychosis

SIDE EFFECTS

Myelosuppression
Dizziness, drowsiness
Hepatitis
Diplopia, rash
Renal failure
Photosensitivity

Nausea, vomiting
Dysrhythmias
Impotence
Bone marrow suppression
Osteoporosis
Hypocholesterolemia

NURSING CONSIDERATIONS

- Take with food or milk to decrease GI upset; nonextended-release tablets may be crushed, extended-release capsules may be opened and mixed with juice or soft food
- Avoid activities requiring alertness for the first 3 days
- Urine may turn pink to brown
- Avoid abrupt withdrawal; discontinue gradually
- Avoid use with alcohol, CNS depressants
- Monitor for suicidal thoughts or behavior
- Patient should wear medical information tag
- Rx

• •

SIDE EFFECTS

Signs of toxicity:
  vomiting,
  diarrhea,
  drowsiness,
  muscular
  weakness, ataxia

Dizziness, headache
Impaired vision
Fine hand tremors
Reversible
  leukocytosis
Dry mouth, anorexia

Hypotension
Dysrhythmias
Polyuria, proteinuria
Hyponatremia
Hypo/
  hyperthyroidism

NURSING CONSIDERATIONS

- Use caution in potentially hazardous activities
- Check serum levels twice weekly during treatment, q 2–3 months on maintenance; draw blood in a.m. prior to dose
- Target serum levels: treatment = 0.5 to 1.5 mEq/L, maintenance = 0.6–1.2 mEq/L
- Take with meals to avoid GI upset
- Onset of therapeutic effects in 1–2 weeks
- Dose reduced during depressive stages of illness
- Encourage 10–12 glasses water/day and adequate salt intake (6–10 g/day)
- Rx

TEMAZEPAM
(tem-<u>az</u>-uh-pam)

(Restoril)

Purpose: short-term treatment of insomnia

. . . .

ZALEPLON
(<u>zall</u>-uh-plon)

(Sonata)

Purpose: short-term treatment of insomnia

SIDE EFFECTS

Drowsiness

Dizziness, headache

Lethargy, fatigue

Weakness

Euphoria

Chest pain, hypotension

Blurred vision

Nausea, vomiting, anorexia

NURSING CONSIDERATIONS

- Should be avoided in patients under the age of 18
- Avoid alcohol while taking this drug
- Not intended for use for more than 10 days
- Take without regard to food
- Increases the effect of CNS depressants
- "Sleep driving" may occur, especially if taken with alcohol or CNS depressants
- Rx C-IV

• •

SIDE EFFECTS

Headache, tremors

Myalgia

Dizziness, confusion

Bronchitis

Dyspepsia, dry mouth

Eye pain, vision change

NURSING CONSIDERATIONS

- Elderly patients generally benefit the most
- Because of rapid onset, patients should take immediately before bedtime
- Avoid alcohol while using this medication
- May be habit-forming
- "Sleep driving" may occur
- Rx C-IV

ZOLPIDEM TARTRATE
(<u>zol</u>-pi-dem)

(Ambien)

Purpose: short-term treatment of insomnia

· ·

Musculoskeletal Medications
Antigout Agents

ALLOPURINOL
(al-oh-<u>pure</u>-i-nole)

(Aloprim, Zyloprim)

Purpose: treatment of gout, hyperuricemia, and uric acid calculi

SIDE EFFECTS

Headache	"Drugged" feeling
Drowsiness	Abnormal thinking
Dizziness	Leukopenia
Nausea	Myalgia

NURSING CONSIDERATIONS

- Dosage may need to be reduced in patient using a CNS depressant, to avoid an addictive effect
- Side effects increase with prolonged usage
- May cause "sleep driving"
- May worsen depression
- Monitor for suicidal thoughts or behavior
- Rx C-IV

• •

SIDE EFFECTS

GI upset
Rash
Malaise

NURSING CONSIDERATIONS

- Encourage 10–12 glasses water/day
- Check CBC, renal and liver function tests before treatment
- Take with food; don't take vitamin C or iron
- Initial therapy can increase attacks of gout
- Avoid use of alcohol, eating organ meats, gravy, legumes
- Full therapeutic effect may require several months
- Management of patients with leukemia, lymphoma who are receiving chemotherapy that may increase uric acid
- Rx

COLCHICINE
(<u>kol</u>-chi-seen)

(Colcrys)

Purpose: prevention and treatment of gouty arthritis; treatment of gout and Mediterranean fever

• •

PROBENECID
(proe-<u>ben</u>-e-sid)

(Probalan)

Purpose: treatment of hyperuricemia in gout and gouty arthritis, adjunct to penicillin treatment

SIDE EFFECTS

Signs of toxicity: abdominal cramp, weakness, nausea, vomiting

Agranulocytosis

Hematuria
Renal damage
Chills, dermatitis
Diarrhea

NURSING CONSIDERATIONS

- Has analgesic, anti-inflammatory effects
- May be taken without regard to meals
- IV: infuse slowly; do not administer IM/subQ
- Encourage 10–12 glasses water/day
- Avoid grapefruit products, alcohol, organ meats, gravy, legumes
- Rx

• •

SIDE EFFECTS

Nausea
Anorexia
Apnea
Hyperglycemia

Skin rash
Hemolytic anemia
Drowsiness, headache

Hypokalemia
Bradycardia
Hepatic necrosis
Nephrotic syndrome

NURSING CONSIDERATIONS

- Give with milk, food, and antacids
- Encourage 8–10 glasses water/day
- Avoid alcohol, organ meats, gravy, legumes
- Avoid aspirin-containing products; may take acetaminophen
- Rx

ADALIMUMAB
(ay-duh-<u>lim</u>-yoo-mab)

(Humira)

Purpose: management of rheumatoid arthritis, psoriatic arthritis, Crohn disease, plaque psoriasis, ankylosing spondylitis, and ulcerative colitis

• •

DICLOFENAC NA
(dye-<u>kloe</u>-fen-ak)

(Voltaren)

Purpose: management of rheumatoid arthritis, osteoarthritis, and dysmenorrhea

SIDE EFFECTS

Headache
Hypertension, CHF
Sinusitis
GI bleeding
Abdominal pain, nausea
Hepatic damage

Leukopenia
Flulike symptoms
Increased cancer risk
UTI
URI, bronchitis

NURSING CONSIDERATIONS

- Treat latent tuberculosis before initiating therapy
- May reactivate hepatitis B in chronic carriers
- Rx

• •

SIDE EFFECTS

Dizziness, drowsiness
Blood dyscrasias
Headache
Nephrotoxicity
Hepatotoxicity

GI distress, bleeding, or ulcer
Rash
Heart failure
Dysrhythmias
MI/stroke

Hearing loss, blurred vision
Photosensitivity
Hyperglycemia

NURSING CONSIDERATIONS

- PO: take with full glass of water and food and remain upright for 30 minutes
- If dose missed, take within 2 hours
- Use with NSAIDs increases anticoagulant effects
- Rx

ETANERCEPT
(eh-<u>tan</u>-ur-sept)

(Enbrel)

Purpose: management of acute chronic rheumatoid arthritis, ankylosing spondylitis, and plaque psoriasis

• •

INDOMETHACIN
(in-doe-<u>meth</u>-a-sin)

(Indocin)

Purpose: treatment of rheumatoid arthritis, osteoarthritis, bursitis, tendinitis, acute gouty arthritis, and ankylosing spondylitis

SIDE EFFECTS

Headache	Dyspepsia	Anemia, leukopenia
Dizziness	Heart failure	URI, cough
Abdominal pain	Hepatitis	

NURSING CONSIDERATIONS

- Instruct patient or caregiver to administer subQ injection
- Do not take live viruses during treatment
- Must be continued for prescribed time to be effective
- Rx

• •

SIDE EFFECTS

Peptic ulcer	Drowsiness	Hepatitis
Dizziness, headache	Nausea, constipation	Blood dyscrasias
Blurred vision	Dysrhythmias	Nephrotoxicity
Tinnitus	MI/stroke	
Hypertension	GI bleeding	

NURSING CONSIDERATIONS

- PO: take with food/milk, encourage upright position for 15–30 minutes
- Use caution with potentially hazardous activities
- Avoid use with alcohol, aspirin, other NSAIDs
- Rx

PIROXICAM
(peer-<u>ox</u>-i-kam)

(Feldene)

Purpose: relief of mild to moderate pain in osteoarthritis and rheumatoid arthritis

• •

SALSALATE
(<u>sal</u>-suh-late)

(Disalcid)

Purpose: relief of mild to moderate pain in osteoarthritis and rheumatoid arthritis

SIDE EFFECTS

Drowsiness, dizziness

Nausea, vomiting

Blurred vision, tinnitus

GI disturbance, bleeding, or ulcer

Rash

Exacerbation of angina

Anemia, leukopenia

Photosensitivity

Hypo/hyperglycemia

Renal failure

Bronchospasms

NURSING CONSIDERATIONS

- PO: with food to decrease GI upset; on empty stomach to increase absorption
- Take at same time every day
- Full therapeutic effect may take up to 1 month for arthritis
- Avoid concurrent use of ASA, OTC meds, alcohol
- Rx

• •

SIDE EFFECTS

Nausea, vomiting

GI bleeding

Vertigo

Heartburn

Rash

Tinnitus

Hearing loss

NURSING CONSIDERATIONS

- PO: can be crushed or taken whole
- PO: take with food or milk to decrease GI upset
- Full therapeutic effect may take 2 weeks
- Do not take another salicylate (ASA) while on this med
- Rx

BACLOFEN
(<u>bak</u>-loe-fen)

(Lioresal)

Purpose: reduction of spasticity in spinal cord injuries and multiple sclerosis

• •

CARISOPRODOL
(kar-eye-soe-<u>proe</u>-dole)

(Soma)

Purpose: relief of pain and stiffness in musculoskeletal disorders

SIDE EFFECTS

Drowsiness

Dizziness

Weakness, fatigue

Confusion

Nausea, vomiting

Headache

Seizures

Hypotension

Chest pain, palpitations

Blurred vision

Respiratory failure

Urinary frequency

NURSING CONSIDERATIONS

- Take with food to decrease GI symptoms
- Avoid alcohol, CNS depressants
- Increased risk of seizures in patients with seizure disorder
- Withdraw gradually over 1 to 2 weeks, unless severe adverse reactions; D/C may cause hallucinations, tachycardia, or rebound spasticity
- Rx

• •

SIDE EFFECTS

Drowsiness

Headache

Insomnia

Dizziness

Nausea

Postural hypotension

Diplopia

Asthma attacks

Eosinophilia

Rash

NURSING CONSIDERATIONS

- PO: onset 30 minutes, peak 4 hours, duration 4–6 hours
- Avoid alcohol, CNS depressants, including OTC cold or allergy meds
- Avoid activities requiring alertness until effects of medication are known
- May cause dependence; use for short term (2–3 weeks)
- Rx C-IV

CYCLOBENZAPRINE
(sye-kloe-<u>ben</u>-za-preen)

(Flexeril)

Purpose: relief of muscle spasms and pain in musculoskeletal conditions

• •

METAXALONE
(meh-<u>tax</u>-uh-lone)

(Skelaxin)

Purpose: relief of pain associated with musculoskeletal injuries

SIDE EFFECTS

Drowsiness

Dizziness

Fatigue

Rash

Dry mouth

Constipation

Headache

Hepatitis

Postural
  hypotension

Dysrhythmias

Diplopia

Change in libido

NURSING CONSIDERATIONS

- Avoid alcohol, CNS depressants, OTC cold and allergy meds
- Avoid activities requiring alertness until effects of medication are known
- Do not discontinue abruptly, taper over 1–2 weeks
- Give with food to decrease GI upset
- Rx

• •

SIDE EFFECTS

Drowsiness

Nervousness

GI upset

Dizziness

Headache

Irritability

Hepatitis

Rash

NURSING CONSIDERATIONS

- Should be an adjunct to rest and physical therapy
- Avoid alcohol while using this drug
- Use caution when operating machinery
- Rx

METHOCARBAMOL
(meth-oh-<u>kar</u>-ba-mole)

(Robaxin)

Purpose: relief of pain associated with musculoskeletal disorders, adjunct in management of neuromuscular manifestations of tetanus

• •

Neurological Medications
Neurological Medications

BENZTROPINE
(<u>benz</u>-troe-peen)

(Cogentin)

Purpose: treatment of Parkinson symptoms, EPS associated with neuroleptic drugs, and acute dystonic reactions

SIDE EFFECTS

Drowsiness
Light-headedness
Hypotension
Dizziness

Nausea
Metallic taste
Urticaria
Blurred vision

NURSING CONSIDERATIONS

- IM: inject deep into muscle of buttock, rotate sites
- NG tube: crush tablets into fluid
- PO: take with food or milk
- Urine may turn green, black, or brown
- Avoid alcohol, CNS depressants, including OTC cold or allergy meds
- Avoid activities requiring alertness until effects of medication are known
- Monitor IV sites carefully for extravasation
- Rx

· ·

SIDE EFFECTS

Dry mouth
Constipation
Weakness
Tardive dyskinesia

Anxiety, irritability
Dizziness, confusion
Palpitations
Hypotension

Photophobia
Urinary retention
Hyperthermia

NURSING CONSIDERATIONS

- IM/IV: onset 15 minutes, duration 6–10 hours
- PO: onset 1 hour, duration 6–10 hours
- Tablets may be crushed and mixed with food
- Taper med over a week, or withdrawal symptoms: EPS, tremors, insomnia, tachycardia, restlessness
- Avoid hazardous activities until stabilized on med
- Change positions slowly
- Avoid alcohol, antihistamines unless directed by provider
- Rx

CAFFEINE/ERGOTAMINE
(er-<u>got</u>-a-meen)

(Cafergot)

Purpose: treatment and prevention of migraines

• •

CARBIDOPA/LEVODOPA
(kar-bih-<u>doe</u>-pa/<u>leev</u>-oe-doe-pa)

(Sinemet)

Purpose: treatment of Parkinson disease and syndrome

SIDE EFFECTS

Nausea

Tremors, convulsions

Toxic ergotism: nausea, vomiting, diarrhea, dizziness, headache, mental confusion

Irregular heart rate

NURSING CONSIDERATIONS

- Take at onset of pain/during prodromal stage to abort headache
- Lie down in darkened quiet room for several hours
- Avoid grapefruit juice
- Do not smoke or use nicotine
- Rx

• •

SIDE EFFECTS

Twitching	Dark urine/sweat	Hemolytic anemia
Headache, dizziness	Cardiac arrhythmias	Rash
Mental changes: confusion, agitation, mood alterations	Orthostatic hypotension	Increased liver function tests
	Blurred vision	
	Nausea, vomiting	

NURSING CONSIDERATIONS

- Take with food; decreased effect with protein
- Full therapeutic effect may take several months
- Change positions slowly
- May cause false positive for urine ketones
- May cause neuroleptic malignant syndrome
- Rx

DONEPEZIL
(doe-<u>nep</u>-uh-zill)

(Aricept)

Purpose: management of dementia in Alzheimer disease

• •

GALANTAMINE, RIVASTIGMINE
(ga-<u>lan</u>-ta-meen, ri-va-<u>stig</u>-meen)

(Razadyne, Exelon)

Purpose: treatment of dementia in mild to moderate Alzheimer disease

SIDE EFFECTS

Nausea, vomiting, diarrhea

Headache, dizziness

Fatigue

Cardiac arrhythmias

Insomnia

Seizures

Rash

Dark urine/sweat

Mental changes

Hypo/hypertension

GI bleeding

Hyperlipidemia

UTI

URI

NURSING CONSIDERATIONS

- Drug does not cure, but stabilizes or relieves symptoms
- Take at regular intervals
- Take between meals or may be given with meals to decrease GI upset
- Rx

• •

SIDE EFFECTS

Nausea

Vomiting

Diarrhea

URI

Anemia

Bradycardia

Tremors, insomnia

NURSING CONSIDERATIONS

- Galantamine and rivastigmine are cholinesterase inhibitors, which increase acetylcholine in the brain, potentially reducing symptoms of dementia
- Drugs do not cure, but stabilize or relieve symptoms
- Use with caution in patients with liver, bladder, or renal disease
- Rx

LISDEXAMFETAMINE DIMESYLATE
(lis-dex-am-<u>fet</u>-a-meen dye-<u>mes</u>-i-late)

(Vyvanse)

Purpose: treatment of ADHA and binge eating disorder

• •

MEMANTINE HCL
(<u>mem</u>-an-teen)

(Namenda XR)

Purpose: treatment of moderate to severe dementia in Alzheimer disease

SIDE EFFECTS

Insomnia
Irritability, restlessness
Decreased appetite
Dry mouth

Upper abdominal pain
Tachycardia, dysrhythmias
Blurred vision

Diplopia
Change in libido
Anorexia

NURSING CONSIDERATIONS

- For individuals age 6 years through adult; effects have not been studied in the elderly
- Interrupt therapy occasionally to determine if there is recurrence of behavioral symptoms sufficient to require continued therapy
- Children and adolescents: sudden death has been reported in patients with structural cardiac abnormalities or other serious heart problems taking CNS stimulant treatment at usual doses
- Adults: sudden death, stroke, and MI have occurred in adults taking stimulant drugs in ADHD doses
- Rx C-II

• •

SIDE EFFECTS

Headache
Constipation
Confusion

Dizziness
Heart failure
Hypertension

Anemia
Back pain
Cough, dyspnea

NURSING CONSIDERATIONS

- Use with caution in patients with liver, bladder, or renal disease
- Capsules can be opened and contents sprinkled on applesauce for patients who have difficulty swallowing pills
- Rx

SELEGILINE
(se-<u>leh</u>-ji-leen)

(Eldepryl)

Purpose: management of Parkinson disease in patients being treated with levodopa/carbidopa

• •

ZOLMITRIPTAN
(zole-mih-<u>trip</u>-tan)

(Zomig)

Purpose: acute treatment of migraines

SIDE EFFECTS

Dizziness

Photosensitivity

Nausea, diarrhea

Headache

Shortness of breath

Insomnia

Orthostatic
   hypotension

Dysrhythmias

Sexual dysfunction

Diplopia

NURSING CONSIDERATIONS

- Do not use with tricyclics or opioids; do not use with meperidine
- Monitor for signs of toxicity: twitching, eye spasms
- Do not stop abruptly; parkinsonian crisis may occur
- Avoid foods high in tyramine (cheese, pickled products), alcohol, large amounts of caffeine
- Rx

• •

SIDE EFFECTS

Weakness, neck stiffness

Tingling, hot sensation,
   burning, feeling of pressure,
   tightness

Numbness, dizziness, sedation

Palpitations, chest pain

Abdominal discomfort

Dyspepsia

Dry mouth

NURSING CONSIDERATIONS

- Take as soon as symptoms occur
- Avoid foods high in tyramine (cheese, pickled products), alcohol, large amounts of caffeine
- May cause serotonin syndrome when used with antidepression medication
- Rx

DORZOLAMIDE HCL
(dor-<u>zoh</u>-la-mide)

(Trusopt)

Purpose: treatment of ocular hypertension and glaucoma

. . . .

LATANOPROST
(luh-<u>tan</u>-uh-prost)

(Xalatan)

Purpose: treatment of glaucoma and ocular hypertension

SIDE EFFECTS

Ocular burning, stinging, discomfort

Blurred vision, tearing, or dryness

Photophobia

Bitter taste in mouth

NURSING CONSIDERATIONS

- Wash hands before and after instillation
- Do not touch tip of dropper to eye or body
- Do not wear contact lenses during instillation
- Drug is a sulfonamide; although given topically, it can be absorbed systemically
- Rx

• •

SIDE EFFECTS

Iris color change

Visual disturbances

Foreign body sensation

Eye discomfort, pain

Angina

NURSING CONSIDERATIONS

- For patients who do not respond to other IOP-lowering drugs
- Wash hands before and after instillation
- Do not touch tip of dropper to eye or body
- Remove contact lenses to give med; can reinsert in 15 minutes
- Rx

TRAVOPROST
(<u>trav</u>-oh-prahst)

(Travatan)

Purpose: treatment of glaucoma and ocular hypertension

• •

LEVOBUNOLOL
(lee-voe-<u>byoo</u>-no-lole)

(AK-Beta, Betagan)

Purpose: treatment of glaucoma and ocular hypertension

SIDE EFFECTS

Ocular hyperemia
Decreased visual acuity
Eye discomfort or pain

Foreign-body sensation
Eye pruritus

NURSING CONSIDERATIONS

- For patients who cannot tolerate or respond inadequately to other IOP-lowering drugs
- Place pressure on tear ducts for 1 minute to avoid systemic absorption
- Wash hands before and after instillation
- Do not touch tip of dropper to eye or body
- Potential for increased brown pigmentation of iris, eyelid skin darkening, changes in eyelashes; important if only one eye is being treated
- Remove contact lenses to give med; can reinsert in 15 minutes
- Discard med 6 months after opening
- Rx

• •

SIDE EFFECTS

Hypotension
Transient eye stinging and
  burning

Palpitations
Insomnia, headache
Bronchospasm

NURSING CONSIDERATIONS

- Place pressure on tear ducts for 1 minute to decrease systemic absorption
- Wash hands before and after instillation
- Do not touch tip of dropper to eye or body
- Drug is a beta blocker
- Report shortness of breath, chest pain, or heart irregularity
- May cause thyroid storm in patients with hypothyroidism
- Rx

TIMOLOL
(<u>tim</u>-oh-lole)

(Timoptic, Betimol solution)

Purpose: treatment of glaucoma and ocular hypertension

• •

BRIMONIDINE TARTRATE
(brih-<u>moh</u>-nih-deen)

(Alphagan P)

Purpose: treatment of glaucoma and ocular hypertension

SIDE EFFECTS

Fatigue	Burning and	Heart failure
Weakness	stinging of eye	Bronchospasm
Hypotension	Palpitations	

NURSING CONSIDERATIONS

- Place pressure on tear ducts for 1 minute to decrease systemic absorption
- Wash hands before and after instillation
- Do not touch drug container to eye or body
- Rx

● ●

SIDE EFFECTS

Pruritus	Visual disturbance
Cough, dyspnea	Eye stinging/burning
Fatigue	Photophobia
Hypertension	Hypercholesterolemia

NURSING CONSIDERATIONS

- Wait 15 minutes after use to wear soft contact lenses
- Use caution with hazardous activities due to decreased mental alertness
- Avoid alcohol
- Monitor intraocular pressure because may reverse after 1 month of therapy
- Wash hands before and after instillation
- Rx

CROMOLYN NA
(<u>kroe</u>-moe-lin)

(Opticrom)

Purpose: relief of itching, burning, and redness of the eyes related to allergy symptoms

• •

TOBRAMYCIN/DEXAMETHASONE
(toe-bruh-<u>mye</u>-sin/dex-uh-<u>meth</u>-uh-sone)

(Tobradex)

Purpose: treatment of conjunctivitis

SIDE EFFECTS
Ocular irritation

NURSING CONSIDERATIONS
- Wash hands before and after instillation
- Do not touch tip of dropper to eye or body
- Do not wear soft contact lenses while using this medication
- Rx

• •

SIDE EFFECTS
Ocular irritation

NURSING CONSIDERATIONS
- Wash hands before and after instillation
- Do not touch tip of dropper to eye or body
- Do not wear contact lenses while using this medication
- Rx

ANTIPYRINE/BENZOCAINE/ GLYCERIN OTIC SOLUTION

(an-tee-<u>pye</u>-reen/<u>ben</u>-zoe-kane/<u>gli</u>-sa-rin <u>oh</u>-tik)

(Auralgan)

Purpose: relief of pain and inflammation in ear

• •

HYDROCORTISONE/NEOMYCIN/ POLYMYXIN OTIC

(hye-droe-<u>kor</u>-tir-sone/nee-uh-<u>mye</u>-sin/pol-i-<u>mix</u>-in <u>oh</u>-tik)

(Cortisporin)

Purpose: treatment of ear infections

SIDE EFFECTS

Allergic reaction: rash, difficulty breathing

NURSING CONSIDERATIONS

- Suspension: shake well (also comes in solution)
- Can warm up with hands for patient's comfort
- Warn patient not to touch ear with dropper
- Warn patient that drug is for use in ears only
- Do not get in eyes, nose, or mouth
- May place cotton plug moistened with medication in ear canal
- Do not rinse dropper
- Rx

• •

SIDE EFFECTS

Allergic reaction: rash,
  difficulty breathing
Burning

NURSING CONSIDERATIONS

- Warn patient not to touch ear with dropper
- Explain drug is for use in ears only
- Possible cross allergy with kanamycin, paromomycin, streptomycin, and gentamicin
- Rx

MONTELUKAST
(mon-te-<u>lew</u>-kast)

(Singulair)

Purpose: prophylaxis and treatment of asthma and seasonal allergic rhinitis

• •

THEOPHYLLINE
(thee-<u>off</u>-i-lin)

Purpose: treatment of bronchial asthma, bronchospasm of chronic bronchitis, and emphysema

SIDE EFFECTS

Dizziness	GI upset	Nasal congestion
Headache	Thrombocytopenia	Muscle cramps
Cough	Pancreatitis	

NURSING CONSIDERATIONS

- Do not use to treat acute symptoms; use a rapid-acting bronchodilator
- Notify provider of wheezing, respiratory distress
- Full therapeutic effect may take several weeks
- May increase risk of neuropsychiatric events including hallucination, aggression, anxiousness, suicidal behavior and thoughts, and tremor
- Rx

• •

SIDE EFFECTS

Restlessness	Anorexia	SIADH
Palpitations, sinus tachycardia	Vomiting	Flushing
Dizziness	Headache	Hyperglycemia
	Insomnia	Tachypnea

NURSING CONSIDERATIONS

- PO: peak 2 hours; take with full glass of water; best on empty stomach
- Check all OTC and other meds for ephedrine before taking with this med
- Avoid alcohol, caffeine, smoking
- Avoid activities requiring alertness until response to med is known
- Contact provider if toxicity: nausea, vomiting, anxiety, insomnia, convulsions
- Drink 8–10 glasses of fluid per day
- Rx

TIOTROPIUM
(tye-oh-<u>troe</u>-pee-um)

(Spiriva, Spiriva HandiHaler)

*Purpose: prevention of bronchial swelling and bronchospasms
  associated with COPD*

• •

BENZONATATE
(ben-<u>zoe</u>-na-tate)

(Tessalon)

Purpose: treatment of nonproductive cough

SIDE EFFECTS

Oral thrush

Vomiting,
  abdominal pain

Skeletal pain

Pharyngitis

Cough, URI

Depression,
  paresthesia

Chest pain,
  increased heart rate

Dry mouth

Urinary difficulty

NURSING CONSIDERATIONS

- Take once daily
- Oral inhalation: onset 30 minutes, peak 2 hours, duration
  24 hours
- Teach how to correctly use inhaler: insert dry powder capsule
  into inhaler device just before inhalation; do not swallow
  capsules; rinse mouth with water after inhalation (decreases side
  effects)
- Do not use as a rescue inhaler (delayed onset, long duration of
  action)
- Rx

• •

SIDE EFFECTS

Dizziness

Drowsiness

Rash

Sedation, headache

Nausea

Constipation

NURSING CONSIDERATIONS

- PO: onset 15–20 minutes, duration 3–8 hours
- Capsules should be swallowed whole; do not chew, because
  release of med may cause local anesthetic effect and choking
- Avoid activities requiring alertness until response to med is
  known
- Rx

IPRATROPIUM

(eye-pra-<u>troe</u>-pee-um)

(Atrovent)

Purpose: treatment of bronchospasms, COPD, and rhinorrhea

• •

ALBUTEROL SULFATE

(al-<u>byoo</u>-ter-ol)

(Proventil-HFA, ProAir HFA)

Purpose: prevention of exercise-induced asthma, acute bronchospasm, bronchitis, and emphysema

SIDE EFFECTS

Nervousness   Palpitations
Nausea, cramps   Blurred vision
Dry mouth   Headache

NURSING CONSIDERATIONS

- Can use with spacer
- Not for acute bronchospasm needing rapid response
- Teach use of metered dose inhaler: inhale, hold breath, exhale slowly
- Don't mix in nebulizer with cromolyn sodium
- Assess for hypersensitivity, including soy products, atropine, peanuts
- Encourage 10–12 glasses water/day
- Avoid OTC cough/hay-fever medications
- Use caution with hazardous activities
- Rx

• •

SIDE EFFECTS

Tremors, anxiety   Heartburn, nausea   Muscle cramps
Headache   Dry nose   Paradoxical
Tachycardia,   Restlessness,   bronchospasms
  palpitations   insomnia
Hypokalemia   Hypo/hypertension

NURSING CONSIDERATIONS

- Teach patient how to correctly use inhaler
- Monitor for toxicity
- Can use with spacer
- Rx

BUDESONIDE/FORMOTEROL
(byoo-<u>dess</u>-oh-nide/for-<u>mot</u>-ur-all)

(Symbicort)

Purpose: prevention of bronchospasm in asthma and COPD

• •

SALMETEROL
(sal-<u>met</u>-uh-rall)

(Serevent)

Purpose: prevention of exercise-induced bronchospasms, treatment of COPD and asthma

SIDE EFFECTS

Thrush	Back pain
Throat irritation	Headache
Vomiting, abdominal pain	Respiratory infection
Flulike symptoms	

NURSING CONSIDERATIONS

- Not for bronchospasms needing rapid response
- Rinse mouth with water after each use
- Teach proper use of inhaler
- Rx

• •

SIDE EFFECTS

Headache	Nausea, vomiting	Hypo/hypertension
Tremors, anxiety	Cough	Dry nose
Throat irritation	Palpitation,	Paradoxical
Myalgia	dysrhythmias	bronchospasm

NURSING CONSIDERATIONS

- Do not use to treat acute symptoms; do not as a use a rapid-acting bronchodilator
- Contact provider if using more than 4 inhalations of a rapid-acting bronchodilator for 2 or more consecutive days
- Teach patient inhaler setup and use
- Rx

TERBUTALINE SULFATE
(ter-<u>byoo</u>-ta-leen)

(Brethine, Bricanyl)

Purpose: treatment of bronchospasms

• •

GUAIFENESIN
(gwye-<u>fen</u>-uh-sin)

(Robitussin, Mucinex, Mytussin)

Purpose: relief of chest congestion by loosening mucus and bronchial secretions

SIDE EFFECTS

Nervousness
Restlessness
Tremor
Palpations, dysrhythmias

Headache
Hypokalemia
Hyperglycemia
Paradoxical bronchospasms

NURSING CONSIDERATIONS

- Inhalation and subQ used for short-term control; PO as long-term
- PO: take with food to decrease GI upset
- Contact provider if unrelieved shortness of breath
- Do not use OTC meds without contacting provider
- Rx

• •

SIDE EFFECTS

Nausea
Headache
Dizziness
Anorexia

NURSING CONSIDERATIONS

- Increase fluid intake
- Do not crush pills
- Take with full glass of water
- OTC, Rx

CROMOLYN SODIUM
(<u>kroe</u>-moe-lin)

(NasalCrom, Crolom)

Purpose: prophylaxis and treatment of allergic rhinitis and bronchial asthma

• •

DISULFIRAM
(dye-<u>sul</u>-fih-ram)

(Antabuse)

Purpose: treatment of alcoholism

SIDE EFFECTS

Nasal burning and irritation
Headache
Dry mouth

Rash
Bronchospasm

NURSING CONSIDERATIONS

- Available as nasal solutions, nebulizer solution, and PO
- Full therapeutic effect may take several weeks
- PO: take 30 minutes before meals, do not crush
- Not appropriate for acute asthma
- Rx

• •

SIDE EFFECTS

In the absence of alcohol: drowsiness, headache, restlessness, fatigue
In the presence of alcohol: flushing, chest pain, heart arrhythmias,
  hypotension, seizures, throbbing in head and neck, sweating

NURSING CONSIDERATIONS

- Causes severe hypersensitivity
- Onset may be delayed up to 12 hours; single dose may be
  effective for 1–2 weeks
- Avoid alcohol in any form: in foods, sauces, or other meds, such
  as cough syrups or tonics
- Avoid vinegar, paregoric, skin products, liniments, or lotions
  containing alcohol
- Do not begin treatment for at least 12 hours after drinking
  alcohol
- Rx

EPOETIN ALFA
(i-<u>poe</u>-uh-tin)

(Epogen)

Purpose: treatment of anemia

• •

Treatment/Replacement
Hair Growth

MINOXIDIL (TOPICAL)
(mi-<u>nox</u>-i-dill)

(Rogaine)

Purpose: treatment of alopecia

SIDE EFFECTS

Headache, fatigue

Coldness, sweating

Hypertension

Hypertensive encephalopathy,
   CHR

Pruritus

Bone pain

Cough

Seizures

NURSING CONSIDERATIONS

- subQ: do not shake vial
- IV: do not dilute or administer with other solutions
- Avoid driving and or hazardous activities during beginning of treatment
- Therapeutic response occurs within 2–4 weeks
- Rx

• •

SIDE EFFECTS

Edema

Increase in body hair

Rash

Headache, fatigue

NURSING CONSIDERATIONS

- Do not use on children or infants
- Avoid contact with eyes, mucous membranes, or sensitive skin areas
- Increasing dosage does not speed growth
- Treatment must continue for long-term
- OTC, Rx

CARBONYL IRON
(<u>kar</u>-buh-nill)

*Purpose: treatment of iron deficiency anemia, prophylaxis for iron
deficiency in pregnancy*

• •

FERRIC GLUCONATE COMPLEX
(<u>fair</u>-ik <u>gloo</u>-kuh-nate)

(Ferrlecit)

Purpose: treatment of iron deficiency anemia in dialysis patients

SIDE EFFECTS

Nausea, constipation
Epigastric pain
Black or discolored stools

NURSING CONSIDERATIONS

- Contains 100% elemental iron
- Keep patient upright for 15–30 minutes to avoid esophageal corrosion; take 1 hour before bedtime
- Stools will become black or dark green
- Notify provider if stools are tarry or blood-streaked; indicates GI bleeding
- Do not substitute one iron salt for another because iron content differs
- Do not take within 1 hour before or 2 hours after antacids, eggs, whole-grain bread or cereal, milk, coffee, or tea
- Liquid may stain teeth
- Rx

• •

SIDE EFFECTS

Hypotension
Flushing

NURSING CONSIDERATIONS

- Given IV
- Notify provider if difficulty breathing or oral edema occurs
- Notify provider if stools are tarry or blood-streaked; indicates GI bleeding
- Do not mix with other medication
- Only mix with 0.9% sodium chloride
- Rx

POTASSIUM CHLORIDE

(puh-<u>tass</u>-ee-um <u>klor</u>-ide)

(K-Tab)

Purpose: prevention and treatment of hypokalemia

• •

NALOXONE HCL

(nal-<u>ox</u>-own)

(Narcan)

Purpose: treatment of respiratory depression induced by opiates

SIDE EFFECTS

Nausea, vomiting
Confusion
Cramps, diarrhea

Cardiac dysrhythmias
Oliguria

NURSING CONSIDERATIONS

- PO: onset 30 minutes; remain upright for 30 minutes after administration
- IV: onset immediate
- Do not infuse faster than 10 mg/hour in adults
- Do not give IM, subQ, IV push
- Dilute liquid prior to giving via NG
- Monitor IV infusions for extravasation: IV infusions may sting or burn
- Report hyperkalemia: lethargy, confusion, GI symptoms, fainting, decreased urinary output
- Avoid OTC antacids, salt substitutes, analgesics, vitamins unless directed by provider
- OTC, Rx

• •

SIDE EFFECTS

Nervousness
Tremor
Rapid pulse

Nausea, vomiting
Dyspnea

NURSING CONSIDERATIONS

- IM and subQ onset in 2–5 minutes; IV 1–2 minutes
- Have emergency support equipment available
- Monitor for bleeding in surgical and obstetric patients
- Withdrawal symptoms in narcotic-dependent patients: restlessness, muscle spasms, tearing
- Rx

ERGOCALCIFEROL
(<u>er</u>-goe-kal-<u>sif</u>-uh-role)

(Vitamin D2)

Purpose: treatment of vitamin D deficiency, rickets, osteomalacia, osteoporosis, and hypoparathyroidism

• •

CYANOCOBALAMIN
(<u>sye</u>-an-oh-koe-<u>bal</u>-a-min)

(Vitamin B12)

Purpose: treatment of vitamin B12 deficiency, pernicious anemia, hemorrhage, and renal and hepatic disease

SIDE EFFECTS

Metallic taste, dry mouth
Hypervitaminosis D

Headache
Fatigue, weakness
Nephrotoxicity

Hypertension
Photophobia

NURSING CONSIDERATIONS

- If med is missed, omit
- Avoid use of antacids and laxatives containing magnesium
- Mineral oil interferes with absorption
- Rx

• •

SIDE EFFECTS

Diarrhea
Hypokalemia
Pulmonary edema
Itching

NURSING CONSIDERATIONS

- IM, subQ, nasal: peak 3–10 days
- Meats, seafood, egg yolk, fermented cheeses are good dietary sources of vitamin B12
- May take with fruit juice to disguise taste
- OTC, Rx

FOLIC ACID
(<u>foe</u>-lik)

Purpose: treatment of anemia, hepatic disease, alcoholism, hemolysis, and intestinal obstruction; reduction of embryonic neural tube defects

• •

Treatment/Replacement

Vitamins

HYDROXOCOBALAMIN
(hye-<u>drox</u>-o-ko-<u>bal</u>-a-min)
(Vitamin B12)

Purpose: treatment of vitamin B12 deficiency, pernicious anemia, malabsorption syndrome, hemolytic anemia, and renal and hepatic disease

SIDE EFFECTS

Bronchospasm
Conduction, irritability
Anorexia

Bitter taste
Pruritus

NURSING CONSIDERATIONS

- Bran, yeast, dried beans, nuts, fruits, fresh vegetables, asparagus are good dietary sources of iron
- May cause urine to turn bright yellow
- OTC

. . . .

SIDE EFFECTS

Diarrhea
Flushing
Pulmonary edema

Hypokalemia
Itching at injection site

NURSING CONSIDERATIONS

- IM, subQ: peak 3–10 days
- Meats, seafood, egg yolk, fermented cheeses are good dietary sources of vitamin B12
- OTC, Rx

DTAP VACCINE
(<u>dee</u>-tap vak-<u>seen</u>)

(Infanrix, Tripedia, Daptacel)

Purpose: prevention of diphtheria, tetanus, and acellular pertussis (whooping cough)

• •

HAEMOPHILUS INFLUENZAE TYPE B (HIB) VACCINE
(hee-<u>mah</u>-fill-us in-floo-<u>en</u>-zee)

(ActHib, PedVaxHib, Hiberix)

Purpose: prevention of Haemophilus influenzae *type B infection*

SIDE EFFECTS

Fever (25%)
Redness or swelling at injection
  site (25%)
Soreness at injection site (25%)

Fussiness (33%)
Serious allergic reaction in less
  than 1 per 1 million doses

NURSING CONSIDERATIONS

- Contains only portions of the bacteria; cannot cause infection
- Control fever with aspirin-free pain reliever, esp. in child with
  seizures
- Children: administer in 5 doses

• •

SIDE EFFECTS

Injection site redness, warmth (uncommon)
Dizziness, shoulder pain (very rare)

NURSING CONSIDERATIONS

- Contains only portions of the bacteria; cannot cause infection
- Children: administer in 3 or 4 doses (depends on brand)

HEPATITIS A VACCINE
(hep-uh-<u>tye</u>-tis aay vak-<u>seen</u>)
(Vaqta, Havrix)

Purpose: prevention of hepatitis A infection

• •

HEPATITIS B VACCINE
(hep-uh-<u>tye</u>-tis bee vak-<u>seen</u>)
(Recombivax HB, Engerix)

Purpose: prevention of hepatitis B infection

SIDE EFFECTS

Soreness at injection site
(50% in adults, 17% in
children)

Headache (17% in adults, 4% in
children)
Serious allergic reaction rare

NURSING CONSIDERATIONS

- Contains the whole, but killed virus; cannot cause infection
- 2 doses needed for lasting protection

● ●

SIDE EFFECTS

Soreness at injection site (25%)
Severe allergic reaction in 1 per 1.1 million doses

NURSING CONSIDERATIONS

- Contains only portions of virus; cannot cause infection
- Infants: administer in 3 doses

HUMAN PAPILLOMAVIRUS (HPV) VACCINE

(<u>hyoo</u>-man pap-ill-<u>oh</u>-mah-<u>vye</u>-rus vak-<u>seen</u>)

(Cervarix for women, Gardasil for both men and women)

Purpose: prevention of infection with HPV types 6, 11, 16, and 18, which cause cervical cancer

• •

INFLUENZA VACCINE

(in-floo-<u>en</u>-zuh vak-<u>seen</u>)

(Fluzone, Flumist nasal spray)

Purpose: prevention of seasonal flu infection

SIDE EFFECTS

Pain at injection site (90% for
  Cervarix, 80% for Gardasil)
Redness or swelling (50% for
  Cervarix, 25% for Gardasil)
Headache or fatigue (50% for
  Cervarix, 33% for Gardasil)

GI symptoms (25% for
  Cervarix)
Muscle or joint pain (50% for
  Cervarix)

NURSING CONSIDERATIONS

- Contains only portions of the virus; cannot cause infection
- Cervarix recommended for girls age 11–12; Gardasil
  recommended for girls and boys age 11–12
- Given as 3-dose series

• •

SIDE EFFECTS

Injection-site swelling, soreness
Flulike symptoms (nasal spray)

NURSING CONSIDERATIONS

- IM: injection contains the whole but killed virus; cannot cause
  infection
- Nasal spray: contains live, weakened viruses; designed to trigger
  a mild infection, inducing immunity
- Serious allergic reaction in less than 1 per 1 million doses

MEASLES, MUMPS, & RUBELLA (MMR) VACCINE
(<u>mee</u>-zulls mumps and roo-<u>bell</u>-uh vak-<u>seen</u>)

(M-M-R II)

Purpose: prevention of infection with measles, mumps, and rubella ("German measles")

• •

MENINGOCOCCAL VACCINE
(men-<u>ing</u>-guh-<u>cok</u>-ull vak-<u>seen</u>)

(Menactra, Menveo)

Purpose: prevention of meningitis infection

SIDE EFFECTS

Fever (17%)

NURSING CONSIDERATIONS

- Contains live but weakened viruses; can cause the actual diseases
- Serious allergic reactions in less than 1 in 1 million doses
- Children: administer in 2 doses

• •

SIDE EFFECTS

Redness or pain at injection site (50%)

NURSING CONSIDERATIONS

- Contains only portions of the bacteria; cannot cause infection
- Adolescents: 2 doses recommended
- Serious allergic reactions very rare

PNEUMOCOCCAL CONJUGATE (PCV13) VACCINE
(<u>new</u>-moe-cok-ull <u>con</u>-juh-get vak-<u>seen</u>)

(Prevnar)

Purpose: prevention of infections caused by Streptococcus
pneumoniae

• •

POLIO VACCINE
(<u>poe</u>-lee-oh vak-<u>seen</u>)

(IPOL)

Purpose: prevention of polio infection

SIDE EFFECTS

Children: drowsiness, anorexia, injection-site redness or tenderness (50%)

Children: irritability (80%)

Children: mild fever, swelling at injection site (33%)

Adults: mild reactions

NURSING CONSIDERATIONS

- PCV13 vaccine protects against 13 of the more than 90 types of pneumococcal bacteria
- PPSV23 vaccine (given to adults over age 65) protects against 23 strains of pneumococcal bacteria
- Contains only portions of the bacteria; cannot cause disease

• •

SIDE EFFECTS

Mild fever

Injection-site soreness

Extremely small risk of allergic reaction

NURSING CONSIDERATIONS

- Contains whole but killed virus; cannot cause disease
- Children: administer in 4 doses

ROTAVIRUS VACCINE
(<u>row</u>-tuh-vye-rus vak-<u>seen</u>)

(Rotateq, Rotarix)

Purpose: prevention of rotavirus infection

. . . .

VARICELLA VACCINE
(<u>vair</u>-i-sell-ah vak-<u>seen</u>)

(Varivax for childhood disease, Zostavax for shingles)

Purpose: prevention of varicella-zoster (chickenpox) infection

SIDE EFFECTS

Irritability
GI upset

NURSING CONSIDERATIONS

- Contains the whole live virus; designed to trigger low-grade infection to create immunity
- Administer PO: oral liquid vaccine
- Infants: administer in 2 or 3 doses (depends on brand)

• •

SIDE EFFECTS

Soreness at injection site
Fever
Rash (rare)

NURSING CONSIDERATIONS

- Both injections contain live, but weakened virus; immunization can cause a mild case of the disease
- Counsel patient to avoid contact with newborns, pregnant women, and immunocompromised individuals immediately after injection

DESOGESTREL/ ETHINYL ESTRADIOL

(des-uh-<u>jes</u>-trul/eh-<u>thye</u>-nul es-truh-<u>dye</u>-ol)

(Desogen, Mircette, Ortho-Cept)

Purpose: contraception, treatment of acne

• •

DROSPIRENONE/ ETHINYL ESTRADIOL

(drah-<u>speer</u>-uh-noan/eh-<u>thye</u>-nul es-truh-<u>dye</u>-ol)

(Yaz)

Purpose: contraception, treatment of acne

SIDE EFFECTS

Headache

Breakthrough
bleeding,
spotting

Contact lens
intolerance

Dizziness

Nausea

Increased clotting
factor

Increased BP

NURSING CONSIDERATIONS

- Monophasic oral contraceptive
- Take at same time each day
- Counsel patient to contact provider if unusual bleeding, severe headache, difficulty breathing, changes in vision/coordination, chest/leg pain
- Counsel patient this medication does not protect against STDs or HIV
- Avoid smoking, which increases risk of adverse cardiovascular events
- St. John's wort and antibiotics may decrease effectiveness
- Rx

• •

SIDE EFFECTS

Headache

Vaginal itching,
discharge, or yeast
infection

Nausea

Breakthrough
bleeding

Increase in BP

Weight gain

Symptoms of
depression

NURSING CONSIDERATIONS

- Monophasic oral contraceptive
- Take at the same time daily, once a day
- Avoid smoking, which increases risk of adverse cardiovascular events
- Counsel patient this medication does not protect against STDs or HIV
- Teach patient to promptly report any visual disturbances, unusual bleeding, chest or leg pain, change in coordination, dyspnea, or severe headache
- May increase risk of cardiovascular events including MI and stroke
- St. John's wort and antibiotics may decrease effectiveness
- Rx

ETHINYL ESTRADIOL/ ETHYNODIOL
(eh-<u>thye</u>-nul es-truh-<u>dye</u>-ol/<u>eth</u>-i-noe-<u>dye</u>-ol)

(Demulen)

Purpose: contraception, treatment of acne

• •

ETHINYL ESTRADIOL/ NORETHINDRONE
(eh-<u>thye</u>-nul es-truh-<u>dye</u>-ol/nor-<u>eth</u>-in-drone)

(Ortho-Novum 7-7-7)

Purpose: contraception, treatment of acne

SIDE EFFECTS

Headache
Breakthrough bleeding,
  spotting

Dizziness
Nausea
Contact lens intolerance

NURSING CONSIDERATIONS

- Monophasic oral contraceptive
- Take at same time each day
- Counsel patient this medication does not protect against STDs or HIV
- Contact provider if unusual bleeding, severe headache, difficulty breathing, changes in vision/coordination, chest/leg pain
- Avoid smoking, which increases risk of adverse cardiovascular events
- Stop med for at least 1 week before surgery to decrease risk of thromboembolism
- St. John's wort and antibiotics may decrease effectiveness
- Rx

• •

SIDE EFFECTS

Nausea
Headache
Breakthrough bleeding

Contact lens intolerance
Dizziness

NURSING CONSIDERATIONS

- Triphasic oral contraceptive
- Take at same time each day
- Counsel patient this medication does not protect against STDs or HIV
- Contact provider if breast lumps, vaginal bleeding, edema, jaundice, dark urine, clay-colored stools, dyspnea, headache, blurred vision, abdominal pain, numbness or stiffness in legs, chest pain, tenderness with redness and swelling in extremities
- Contact provider if weekly weight gain is over 5 pounds
- Can take with food or milk to decrease GI upset
- St. John's wort and antibiotics may decrease effectiveness
- Rx

MESTRANOL/ NORETHINDRONE
(<u>mes</u>-truh-nol/nor-<u>eth</u>-in-drone)

(Norinyl)

Purpose: contraception, treatment of acne and endometriosis

• •

NORETHINDRONE
(nor-<u>eth</u>-in-drone)

(Micronor, Nor-Qd, Nor-QD)

Purpose: contraception, treatment of abnormal bleeding and endometriosis

SIDE EFFECTS

Headache

Breakthrough bleeding,
  spotting

Contact lens intolerance

Dizziness

Nausea

NURSING CONSIDERATIONS

- Monophasic oral contraceptive
- Counsel patient this medication does not protect against STDs
  or HIV
- Contact provider if unusual bleeding, severe headache, difficult
  breathing, changes in vision/coordination, chest/leg pain
- Avoid smoking, which increases risk of adverse cardiovascular
  events
- St. John's wort and antibiotics may decrease effectiveness
- Rx

• •

SIDE EFFECTS

Nausea

Headache

Dizziness

Breakthrough bleeding

NURSING CONSIDERATIONS

- Progestin oral contraceptive
- Counsel patient this medication does not protect against STDs or
  HIV
- Contact provider if breast lumps, vaginal bleeding, edema,
  jaundice, dark urine, clay-colored stools, dyspnea, headache,
  blurred vision, abdominal pain, numbness or stiffness in legs,
  chest pain, tenderness with redness and swelling in extremities
- Contact provider if weekly weight gain is over 5 pounds
- Can take with food or milk to decrease GI upset
- Cigarette smoking increases risk of serious cardiovascular disease
- Rx

ESTRADIOL (ORAL)

(es-truh-<u>dye</u>-ol)

(Estrace)

Purpose: treatment of menopausal symptoms, inoperable breast cancer, prostatic cancer, and atrophic vaginitis; prevention of osteoporosis

• •

ESTRADIOL CYPIONATE, ESTRADIOL VALERATE

(es-truh-<u>dye</u>-ol si-<u>pye</u>-uh-nate, es-truh-<u>dye</u>-ol <u>val</u>-uh-rate)

(Depogen, Delestrogen, Valergen)

Purpose: treatment of menopausal symptoms, inoperable breast cancer, prostatic cancer, and atrophic vaginitis; prevention of osteoporosis

SIDE EFFECTS

Nausea
Gynecomastia
Contact lens
intolerance
Weight gain

Testicular atrophy
Impotence
Headache
Dizziness
Hypertension

Thromboembolism,
MI
Hypercalcemia
Hyperglycemia

NURSING CONSIDERATIONS

- Contact provider if breast lumps, vaginal bleeding, edema, jaundice, dark urine, clay-colored stools, dyspnea, headache, blurred vision, abdominal pain, numbness or stiffness in legs, chest pain, tenderness with redness and swelling in extremities
- Men should contact provider to report impotence or gynecomastia
- Contact provider if weekly weight gain is over 5 pounds
- Can take with food or milk to decrease GI upset
- May increase risk of endometrial cancer and breast cancer
- May increase risk of cardiovascular events
- Rx

• •

SIDE EFFECTS

Contact lens
intolerance
Gynecomastia
Nausea
Testicular atrophy

Impotence
Weight gain
Headache, dizziness
Hypertension

Thromboembolism,
MI
Hypercalcemia
Hyperglycemia

NURSING CONSIDERATIONS

- IM: inject deep into large muscle mass
- Contact provider if breast lumps, vaginal bleeding, edema, jaundice, dark urine, clay-colored stools, dyspnea, headache, blurred vision, abdominal pain, numbness or stiffness in legs, chest pain, tenderness with redness and swelling in extremities
- Men should contact provider to report impotence or gynecomastia
- Contact provider if weekly weight gain is over 5 pounds
- May increase risk of cardiovascular events
- May increase risk of endometrial and breast cancer
- Rx

ESTRADIOL PATCH
(es-truh-<u>dye</u>-ol)

(Alora, Climara, Estraderm, FemPatch)

Purpose: treatment of menopausal symptoms, inoperable breast cancer, prostatic cancer, and atrophic vaginitis; prevention of osteoporosis

• •

ESTROGENS CONJUGATED
(<u>ess</u>-truh-jenz <u>kon</u>-juh-gate-id)

(Premarin)

Purpose: treatment of menopausal symptoms and atrophic vaginitis, palliative therapy for breast cancer and prostatic cancer

SIDE EFFECTS

Contact lens intolerance

Gynecomastia

Testicular atrophy

Impotence

Hypertension

Weight gain

Thromboembolism

Hyperglycemia

Hypercalcemia

NURSING CONSIDERATIONS

- Apply patch to trunk of body twice a week; press firmly and hold in place for 10 seconds to ensure good contact
- Contact provider if breast lumps, vaginal bleeding, edema, jaundice, dark urine, clay-colored stools, dyspnea, headache, blurred vision, abdominal pain, numbness or stiffness in legs, chest pain, tenderness with redness and swelling in extremities
- Men should contact provider to report impotence or gynecomastia
- Contact provider if weekly weight gain is over 5 pounds
- May increase risk of cardiovascular events
- May increase risk of endometrial cancer and breast cancer
- Rx

• •

SIDE EFFECTS

Nausea

Gynecomastia

Contact lens intolerance

Testicular atrophy

Impotence

NURSING CONSIDERATIONS

- IM: inject deep into large muscle mass
- PO: can take with food or milk to decrease GI upset
- Contact provider if breast lumps, vaginal bleeding, edema, jaundice, dark urine, clay-colored stools, dyspnea, headache, blurred vision, abdominal pain, numbness or stiffness in legs, chest pain, tenderness with redness and swelling in extremities
- Men should contact provider to report impotence or gynecomastia
- Contact provider if weekly weight gain is over 5 pounds
- May increase risk of cardiovascular events
- May increase risk of endometrial cancer and ovarian cancer
- Rx

CLOMIPHENE CITRATE
(<u>klo</u>-muh-feen <u>sih</u>-trate)

(Clomid, Serophene)

Purpose: stimulation of ovulation to increase fertility

• •

MEDROXYPROGESTERONE ACETATE
(meh-<u>drox</u>-ee-proe-<u>jess</u>-tuh-rone <u>a</u>-suh-tate)

(Provera, Depo-Provera)

Purpose: contraception; management of uterine bleeding, secondary amenorrhea, endometrial cancer, and renal cancer

SIDE EFFECTS

Vasomotor flushes
Breast discomfort
Heavy menses
Mental depression
Headache
Nausea, vomiting
Constipation, bloating

Spontaneous abortion
Multiple ovulations
Enlarged ovaries with multiple follicular cysts
Ophthalmic "floaters," diplopia

Deep vein thrombosis
Hepatitis

NURSING CONSIDERATIONS

- Teach patient to report abnormal bleeding, pelvic pain, hot flashes immediately
- Patient should stop medication if pregnancy is suspected
- Rx

• •

SIDE EFFECTS

Nausea
Diplopia
Testicular atrophy
Dizziness
Impotence

GI upset
Galactorrhea
Depression
Hyperglycemia
Stroke/MI

Photosensitivity
Decreased bone density

NURSING CONSIDERATIONS

- IM: inject deep into large muscle mass, rotate sites, injection may be painful
- Counsel patient this medication does not protect against STDs or HIV
- Contact provider if weekly weight gain is over 5 pounds
- Contact provider if swelling in calves, sudden chest pain, or SOB
- May increase risk of cardiovascular events
- May increase risk of ovarian and breast cancer
- Rx

APPENDIX A:
Controlled Substance Schedules

Drugs regulated by the Controlled Substances Act of 1970 are classified as follows.

Schedule I: High abuse potential and no accepted medical use. Examples include heroin, marijuana, peyote, Ecstasy, and LSD.

Schedule II: High abuse potential with severe dependence liability. Examples include narcotics, amphetamines, and some barbiturates.

Schedule III: Less abuse potential than schedule II drugs and moderate dependence liability. Examples include nonbarbiturate sedatives, nonamphetamine stimulants, anabolic steroids, and limited amounts of certain narcotics.

Schedule IV: Less abuse potential than schedule III drugs and limited dependence liability. Examples include some sedatives, anxiolytics, and nonnarcotic analgesics.

Schedule V: Limited abuse potential. Examples include small amounts of narcotics, such as codeine, used as antidiarrheals or antitussives.

APPENDIX B:
Special Considerations

Black box warning, also known as boxed warning: Food and Drug Administration (FDA) warning placed by the manufacturer on a prescription drug package insert. It communicates that the medication carries a significant risk of serious or even life-threatening adverse effects.

Off-label use: Use of medications for an unapproved indication or in an unapproved age group, unapproved dosage, or unapproved route of administration.

Pregnancy and lactation: Prior to June 2015, the FDA required that most prescribed medications be labeled for risk according to letter categories A (remote possibility of fetal harm), B, C, D, and X (studies show evidence of fetal risk). Beginning in June 2015, the FDA changed to a system in which health care providers assess the benefit versus the risk of a given medication for individual pregnant women and nursing mothers. FDA guidelines call for subsequent counseling of pregnant and lactating patients, "allowing them to make informed and educated decisions for themselves and their children." The FDA created a pregnancy exposure registry to collect and maintain data on the effects of approved drugs that are prescribed to and used by pregnant women (FDA *Pregnancy and Lactation Labeling Final Rule*, December 3, 2014).

APPENDIX C:

Common Medical Abbreviations

ABC—airway, breathing, circulation

abd.—abdomen

ABG—arterial blood gas

ABO—system of classifying blood groups

ac—before meals

ACE—angiotensin-converting enzyme

ACS—acute compartment syndrome

ACTH—adrenocorticotrophic hormone

ADH—antidiuretic hormone

ADHD—attention deficit hyperactivity disorder

ADL—activities of daily living

ad lib—freely, as desired

AFP—alpha-fetoprotein

AIDS—acquired immunodeficiency syndrome

AKA—above-the-knee amputation

ALL—acute lymphocytic leukemia

ALS—amyotrophic lateral sclerosis

ALT—alanine transaminase (formerly SGPT)

AMI—antibody-mediated immunity

AML—acute myelogenous leukemia

amt.—amount

ANA—antinuclear antibody

ANS—autonomic nervous system

AP—anteroposterior

A&P—anterior and posterior

APC—atrial premature contraction

aq.—water

ARDS—adult respiratory distress syndrome

ASD—atrial septal defect

ASHD—atherosclerotic heart disease

AST—aspartate aminotransferase (formerly SGOT)

ATP—adenosine triphosphate

AV—atrioventricular

BCG—bacille Calmette-Guérin

bid—two times a day

BKA—below-the-knee amputation

BLS—basic life support

BMR—basal metabolic rate

BP—blood pressure

BPH—benign prostatic hypertrophy

bpm—beats per minute

Abbreviations

BPR—bathroom privileges

BSA—body surface area

BUN—blood, urea, nitrogen

C—centigrade, Celsius

c—with

Ca—calcium

CA—cancer

CABG—coronary artery bypass graft

CAD—coronary artery disease

CAPD—continuous ambulatory peritoneal dialysis

caps—capsules

CBC—complete blood count

CC—chief complaint

CCU—coronary care unit, critical care unit

CDC—Centers for Disease Control and Prevention

CHF—congestive heart failure

CK—creatine kinase

Cl—chloride

CLL—chronic lymphocytic leukemia

cm—centimeter

CMV—cytomegalovirus infection

CNS—central nervous system

CO—carbon monoxide, cardiac output

CO$_2$—carbon dioxide

comp—compound

cont—continuous

COPD—chronic obstructive pulmonary disease

CP—cerebral palsy

CPAP—continuous positive airway pressure

CPK—creatine phosphokinase

CPR—cardiopulmonary resuscitation

CRP—C-reactive protein

C&S—culture and sensitivity

CSF—cerebrospinal fluid

CT—computed tomography

CTD—connective tissue disease

CTS—carpal tunnel syndrome

cu—cubic

CVA—cerebrovascular accident or costovertebral angle

CVC—central venous catheter

CVP—central venous pressure

D&C—dilation and curettage

DIC—disseminated intravascular coagulation

DIFF—differential blood count

dil.—dilute

DJD—degenerative joint disease

DKA—diabetic ketoacidosis

dL—deciliter (100 mL)

DM—diabetes mellitus

DNA—deoxyribonucleic acid

DNR—do not resuscitate

DO—doctor of osteopathy

DOE—dyspnea on exertion

DPT—vaccine for diphtheria, pertussis, tetanus

Dr.—doctor

DVT—deep vein thrombosis

D/W—dextrose in water

Dx—diagnosis

ECF—extracellular fluid

ECG or EKG—electrocardiogram

ECT—electroconvulsive therapy

ED—emergency department

EEG—electroencephalogram

EMD—electromechanical dissociation

EMG—electromyography

ENT—ear, nose, and throat

ESR—erythrocyte sedimentation rate

ESRD—end stage renal disease

ET—endotracheal tube

F—Fahrenheit

FBD—fibrocystic breast disease

FBS—fasting blood sugar

FDA—U.S. Food and Drug Administration

FFP—fresh frozen plasma

fl—fluid

4 x 4—piece of gauze 4 inches long by 4 inches wide used for dressings

FSH—follicle-stimulating hormone

ft.—foot, feet (unit of measure)

FUO—fever of undetermined origin

g—gram

GB—gallbladder

GFR—glomerular filtration rate

GH—growth hormone

GI—gastrointestinal

gr—grain

GSC—Glasgow coma scale

GTT—glucose tolerance test

gtts—drops

GU—genitourinary

GYN—gynecological

h or hrs—hour or hours

(H)—hypodermically

Hb or Hgb—hemoglobin

hCG—human chorionic gonadotropin

HCO$_3^-$—bicarbonate

Hct—hematocrit

HD—hemodialysis

HDL—high-density lipoproteins

Hg—mercury

Hgb—hemoglobin

HGH—human growth hormone

HHNC—hyperglycemia hyperosmolar nonketotic coma

HIV—human immunodeficiency virus

HLA—human leukocyte antigen

HR—heart rate

hr—hour

HSV—herpes simplex virus

HTN—hypertension

H₂O—water

Hx—history

Hz—hertz (cycles/second)

IAPB—intraaortic balloon pump

IBS—irritable bowel syndrome

ICF—intracellular fluid

ICP—intracranial pressure

ICS—intercostal space

ICU—intensive care unit

IDDM—insulin-dependent diabetes mellitus

IgA—immunoglobulin A

IM—intramuscular

I&O—intake and output

IOP—intraocular pressure

IPG—impedance plethysmogram

IPPB—intermittent positive-pressure breathing

IUD—intrauterine device

IV—intravenous

IVC—intraventricular catheter

IVP—intravenous pyelogram

JRA—juvenile rheumatoid arthritis

K⁺—potassium

kcal—kilocalorie (food calorie)

kg—kilogram

KO, KVO—keep vein open

KS—Kaposi sarcoma

KUB—kidneys, ureters, bladder

L, l—liter

lab—laboratory

lb—pound

LBBB—left bundle branch block

LDH—lactate dehydrogenase

LDL—low-density lipoproteins

LE—lupus erythematosus

LH—luteinizing hormone

liq—liquid

LLQ—left lower quadrant

LOC—level of consciousness

LP—lumbar puncture

LPN, LVN—licensed practical or vocational nurse

LTC—long-term care

LUQ—left upper quadrant

LV—left ventricle

m—meter, micron

MAOI—monoamine oxidase inhibitor

MAST—military antishock trousers

mcg—microgram

MCH—mean corpuscular hemoglobin

MCV—mean corpuscular volume

MD—muscular dystrophy, medical doctor

MDI—metered dose inhaler

mEq—milliequivalent

mg—milligram

Mg—magnesium

MG—myasthenia gravis

MI—myocardial infarction

mL—milliliter

mm—millimeter

MMR—vaccine for measles, mumps, and rubella

MRI—magnetic resonance imaging

MS—multiple sclerosis

N—nitrogen, normal (strength of solution)

NIDDM—non-insulin-dependent diabetes mellitus

Na+—sodium

NaCl—sodium chloride

NANDA—North American Nursing Diagnosis Association

NG—nasogastric

NGT—nasogastric tube

NLN—National League for Nursing

noc—at night

NPO—nothing by mouth

NS—normal saline

NSR—normal sinus rhythm (cardiac)

NSAIDs—nonsteroidal anti-inflammatory drugs

NSNA—National Student Nurses' Association

NST—nonstress test

O₂—oxygen

OB-GYN—obstetrics and gynecology

OCT—oxytocin challenge test

OOB—out of bed

OPC—outpatient clinic

OR—operating room

os—by mouth

OSHA—Occupational Safety and Health Administration

OTC—over-the-counter (drug that can be obtained without a prescription)

oz—ounce

p—with

P—pulse, pressure, phosphorus

PA chest—posterior-anterior chest x-ray

PAC—premature atrial complexes

PaCO₂—partial pressure of carbon dioxide in arterial blood

PaO₂—partial pressure of oxygen in arterial blood

PAD—peripheral artery disease

Pap—Papanicolaou smear

PBI—protein-bound iodine

pc—after meals

PCA—patient-controlled analgesia

PCO₂—partial pressure of carbon dioxide

PCP—*Pneumocystis jiroveci* pneumonia (formerly *Pneumocystis carinii* pneumonia)

PD—peritoneal dialysis

PE—pulmonary embolism

PEEP—positive end-expiratory pressure

PERRLA—pupils equal, round, reactive to light and accommodation

PET—postural emission tomography

PFT—pulmonary function tests

pH—hydrogen ion concentration

PID—pelvic inflammatory disease

PKD—polycystic disease

PKU—phenylketonuria

PMDD—premenstrual dysphoric disorder

PMS—premenstrual syndrome

PND—paroxysmal nocturnal dyspnea

PO, po—by mouth

PO₂—partial pressure of oxygen

PPD—positive purified protein derivative (of tuberculin)

PPN—partial parenteral nutrition

PRN, prn—as needed, whenever necessary

pro time—prothrombin time

PSA—prostate-specific antigen

psi—pounds per square inch

PSP—phenolsulfonphthalein

PT—physical therapy, prothrombin time

PTCA—percutaneous transluminal coronary angioplasty

PTH—parathyroid hormone

PTT—partial thromboplastin time

PUD—peptic ulcer disease

PVC—premature ventricular contraction

q—every

QA—quality assurance

qh—every hour

q 2 h—every 2 hours

q 4 h—every 4 hours

qid—four times a day

qs—quantity sufficient

R—rectal temperature, respirations, roentgen

RA—rheumatoid arthritis

RAI—radioactive iodine

RAIU—radioactive iodine uptake

RAS—reticular activating system

RBBB—right bundle branch block

RBC—red blood cell or count

RCA—right coronary artery

RDA—recommended dietary allowance

resp—respirations

RF—rheumatic fever, rheumatoid factor

Rh—antigen on blood cell indicated by + or –

RIND—reversible ischemic neurologic deficit

RLQ—right lower quadrant

RN—registered nurse

RNA—ribonucleic acid

R/O, r/o—rule out, to exclude

ROM—range of motion (of joint)

RUQ—right upper quadrant

Rx—prescription

s̄—without

S. or Sig.—(Signa) to write on label

SA—sinoatrial node

SaO$_2$—systemic arterial oxygen saturation (%)

sat sol—saturated solution

SBE—subacute bacterial endocarditis

SDA—same-day admission

SDS—same-day surgery

sed rate—sedimentation rate

SGOT—serum glutamic-oxaloacetic transaminase (see AST)

SGPT—serum glutamic-pyruvic transaminase (see ALT)

SI—International System of Units

SIADH—syndrome of inappropriate antidiuretic hormone

SIDS—sudden infant death syndrome

SL—sublingual

SLE—systemic lupus erythematosus

SOB—short of breath

sol—solution

SMBG—self-monitoring blood glucose

SMR—submucous resection

sp gr—specific gravity

spec.—specimen

SSKI—saturated solution of potassium iodide

stat—immediately

STI—sexually transmitted infection

subcut, subQ—subcutaneous

Sx—symptoms

Syr.—syrup

T—temperature, thoracic (to be followed by the number designating specific thoracic vertebra)

T&A—tonsillectomy and adenoidectomy

tabs—tablets

TB—tuberculosis

T&C—type and crossmatch

Abbreviations

TED—thromboembolic device (compression stockings)

temp—temperature

TENS—transcutaneous electrical nerve stimulation

TIA—transient ischemic attack

TIBC—total iron binding capacity

tid—three times a day

tinct, or tr.—tincture

TMJ—temporomandibular joint

tPA, TPA—tissue plasminogen activator

TPN—total parenteral nutrition

TPR—temperature, pulse, respiration

TQM—total quality management

TSE—testicular self-examination

TSH—thyroid-stimulating hormone

tsp—teaspoon

TSS—toxic shock syndrome

TURP—transurethral prostatectomy

UA—urinalysis

ung—ointment

URI—upper respiratory tract infection

UTI—urinary tract infection

VAD—venous access device

VDRL—Venereal Disease Research Laboratory (test for syphilis)

VF, Vfib—ventricular fibrillation

VPC—ventricular premature complexes

VS, vs—vital signs

VSD—ventricular septal defect

VT—ventricular tachycardia

WBC—white blood cell or count

WHO—World Health Organization

wt—weight

BRAND NAME DRUG INDEX

GENERIC NAME DRUG INDEX